THE NURSE EDUCATOR IN ACADEMIA:
Strategies for Success

Theresa M. Valiga, EdD, RN, received her bachelor's degree in nursing from Trenton State College and her master's and doctor's degrees, both in Nursing Education, from Teachers College, Columbia University. She has been a faculty member at Trenton State College, Seton Hall University, and Georgetown University, and currently holds the position of Associate Professor and Director of the Graduate Program in the College of Nursing at Villanova University. Dr. Valiga's primary research interest relates to student cognitive development. Her publications and presentations center around this topic as well as leadership development, creativity in teaching, and various professional issues.

Helen J. Streubert, EdD, RN, is Assistant Professor and Coordinator of the Home Health Care Clinical Specialist Concentration at Thomas Jefferson University. Dr. Streubert earned her doctor's degree in nursing education from Teachers College, Columbia University. Her master's degree is from Villanova University, and her bachelor's degree is from Cedar Crest College. Dr. Streubert's primary research interest is clinical education of nursing students. She has presented her research in national and international forums.

The Nurse Educator in Academia: Strategies for Success

Theresa M. Valiga,
EdD, RN

Helen J. Streubert,
EdD, RN

SPRINGER PUBLISHING COMPANY · NEW YORK

Springer Publishing Company, Inc.
536 Broadway
New York, NY 10012-3955

91 92 93 94 95 / 5 4 3 2 1

Library of Congress Cataloging-in-Publication Data

Valiga, Theresa M.
    The nurse educator in academia : strategies for success / Theresa
M. Valiga, Helen J. Streubert.
        p.   cm. — (Springer series on the teaching of nursing : v.
13)
    Includes bibliographical references and index.
    ISBN 0-8261-7150-8
    1. Nursing schools — Faculty.   2. Nursing — Vocational guidance.
I. Streubert, Helen J.   II. Title.   III. Series.
    [DNLM: 1. Education, Nursing.   2. Teaching.   W1 SP685SG v. 13 /
WY 18 V172n]
    RT73.V34   1990
    610.73′0711 — dc20
    DNLM/DLC
for Library of Congress   90-10437
                                                            CIP
                                                            Rev.

Printed in the United States of America

To the many faculty colleagues and students I have known over the years, for their role in helping me grow. And to Bob, who is always there to encourage, inspire, believe in, and love me.

T. M. V.

To the three men in my life, Edward, Michael, and Matthew who have always loved me and provided me with the space to be who I want to be.

H. J. S.

Contents

Foreword

Without a guide through the often unstated rules and mores of the academic world, the experience of a new nurse faculty member can often be an isolating one. Sometimes I have an image of nursing faculty as characters in Virginia Woolf's short novel *Between the Acts* (1941) as guests at a garden party on a beautiful estate owned by a woman of privilege and culture. Despite the beauty and culture and privilege of the experience, they are each haunted by a gramophone in the background, which plays and replays throughout the day, the same refrain: "Dispersed are we, we who come together.... All is over. The wave has broken. Left us stranded, high and dry. Single, separate on the shingle" (p. 96).

Consider this book a mentor—your personal guide through what can be a fragmented and disjointed experience. The ideology and structure of the university leads easily to the individual's retreat as the solution to such feelings as Woolf's guests describe. Nurse educators have a long tradition of efforts at community building within their programs: Isabel Stewart for instance, "call[ed] for a more democratic type of leadership which operates through groups rather than through the concentration of power and authority on certain individuals" (Stewart, 1950, p. 383). This book can be seen as part of that tradition. The values of collegiality, shared respect, and concerned relationships are central to nursing. Theresa Valiga and Helen Streubert's book, which is at once both an artfully crafted reference on the faculty's role and a model of the guidance, help, and friendship possible between a junior and senior colleague, is a welcome and significant contribution.

PATRICIA MOCCIA, PHD, RN, FAAN

Introduction

Beginning any new job is a challenging and sometimes frightening experience. When that new job also involves taking on a totally new role, functioning in a unique system, and interacting with professionals from diverse backgrounds and disciplines, it can be even more overwhelming. Such is the case for a new nursing faculty member.

The new nursing faculty member in higher education enters that role with a recognized level of clinical expertise and advanced educational preparation and, frequently, extensive experience in nursing. Typically, that individual's master's preparation has been as a clinical nurse specialist, with a course in teaching methods possibly being included in the program of study. Although this individual has had multiple experiences teaching clients and families in the clinical area, and although he or she may have taken a course in teaching and learning, this often is not enough to prepare one fully for the academic world.

The norms and expectations in academe are different from those in the clinical arena. The responsibilities of a faculty role are different from those of a clinician. The colleagues with whom one interacts are not all health oriented, and many have a limited understanding of nursing, the health care system, and the uniqueness of preparing students for professional practice roles. Thus, the new nurse faculty member must develop new understandings and new "modes of operation."

This book is intended to help new nursing faculty members make the transition in role from that of *nurse* to that of *nurse educator* (Infante, 1986). It has been written by two nurse educators with a total of 26 years of experience in faculty roles, in several different senior colleges and universities as well as junior colleges. The authors were both prepared specifically as nurse educators and yet, they have struggled—through years of experience, continued study, and extensive dialogue—to understand better the faculty role, the academic system, and the issues and problems facing nursing faculty. This book is an attempt to help new faculty members or graduate students intending to pursue a career in academe achieve similar understandings earlier in their careers.

In addition to sharing similar career interests and goals, the authors also share a professional colleagueship and a friendship, both of which evolved from a student-teacher and then a mentor-protégée relationship. Most of the topics and issues addressed in this book were real ones discussed between the two authors as the student-protégée prepared for and then assumed a faculty role and as the teacher-mentor continued her professional development.

As is true for many faculty members, the authors have been challenged by issues such as balancing numerous faculty roles (e.g., teacher, scholar, actively involved professional, author), evaluating students, teaching nontraditional students, undergoing peer review, and preparing for National League for Nursing (NLN) accreditation. They talked about these and other challenges at length, and when life situations changed, they continued this dialogue through letters.

The "Dear Terry/Dear Helen" letters that introduce each of the five units in the book have been written to summarize selected issues about the academic system itself, students, personal advancement, providing quality education, and faculty evaluation. They also were written to reflect the very personal nature of many of these issues—how they can "get under one's skin" and how they can mean so much to an individual—and to reinforce the value of a mentor relationship.

Unit I presents information, issues, and ideas that will help the novice nurse educator enter and understand the academic system. It discusses aspects of finding and securing one's first faculty appointment including the search and interview process, contract negotiations, and the importance of considering one's personal values and professional goals when contemplating a position offer. This unit also presents an overview of the responsibilities of the various individuals with whom a faculty member may interact in carrying out his or her role (e.g., dean, level coordinator, curriculum coordinator) and discusses how nursing is, can be, or should be an integral part of the overall university or college system. The value of nursing on one's campus is addressed as is the faculty role in advancing or promoting nursing on campus. Finally, this unit looks closely at the NLN, how it influences nursing curricula and faculty activities, and how the accreditation process can enable an individual or a group of nursing faculty to achieve their goals.

Unit II offers suggestions on thriving in the academic system. An analysis of the multiple responsibilities of a nurse educator is provided, and the "ins and outs" of the promotion and tenure process are discussed. The issues and questions that work load and professional advancement in academe present to nurse educators are numerous and complex; the discussions offered here may help clarify some of the confusion surrounding these "sacred cows" and assist nurse educators in their quest for advancement within the academic system.

In Unit III the issue of providing quality education is addressed. Quality education is a multifaceted responsibility of many individuals, which reflects a variety of processes and presents many challenges. One of the ways to achieve quality education is to implement the nursing program's philosophy and curriculum model as they have been outlined, and a discussion of how this can be accomplished is offered. Quality education is also achieved through the close collaboration of nurse educators and nursing service providers; common misunderstandings between these two groups are analyzed, and ways to "bridge the gap" between these seemingly divergent subcultures in nursing are suggested. Finally, quality education is accomplished by the advancement and graduation of well-prepared students; thus, the issues of evaluating students and the responsibilities of faculty in this area are discussed thoroughly.

Evaluation is one faculty responsibility that involves students, but several other student-related issues also warrant analysis, and these are presented in Unit IV. Teaching the nontraditional or diverse learner is becoming more and more commonplace for nurse educators, and it is important that faculty members have the understanding and skill needed to work effectively with such students. Nurse educators also must be well aware of the legal aspects of teaching including student rights and the responsibilities they place on faculty, and they must be able to manage the situation successfully when a student fails an assignment or a course—an unfortunate but all-too-real experience for faculty.

Finally, the new nurse educator needs to be informed about the process of faculty evaluation and his or her role in that process. Unit V presents an analysis of the "who, what, where, why, and how" of faculty evaluation, and concludes by relating this process to career development and the enhancement of nursing's effectiveness in the academic community.

Although there are many more aspects of a nurse educator's role and numerous other challenges such a role presents, we hope that the topics discussed here will provide an adequate basis for the new nurse educator or the graduate student. It is through knowledge and self-reflection that we grow and achieve our goals. Our hope is that this book helps nurse educators begin to develop the needed knowledge base, and that it stimulates self-reflection.

REFERENCE

Infante, M.S. (1986). The conflicting roles of the nurse and the nurse educator. *Nurse Outlook, 36*(2), 94–96.

UNIT I
Entering and Understanding the Academic System

LETTERS

Dear Terry,

It is hard to believe that I'm finally here. It's been almost six weeks. I have a real office with a desk and chair, file cabinet, certificates on the wall and a telephone of my own—all of the makings of a bona fide academician. Sitting here I find myself reflecting on how I arrived here. Graduate school had some very comforting assets, the biggest one of them being security. I was very frightened by having to "sell" myself. When I first started looking for a position, I realized that the newspapers and journals were not affording me the opportunities that I knew were out there. I decided that probably the best place to find the *real* information was by going to some local professional organization meetings. I chose the American Nurses Association meetings because a few colleagues from the hospital where I used to work went regularly, and they seemed to have a handle on all of the local openings. I guess I could have just gone to lunch with them, but I really felt the need to get back into professional circles locally. I almost perceived myself as having been in some sort of state of limbo during my time in graduate school.

The interviews that I went on were as much learning experiences as they were job-seeking sessions. It is amazing that all of the different sorts of teaching arrangements, workload formulas, and employment contracts exist. One school offered the opportunity to team teach in an integrated curriculum. When I had the opportunity to meet with a group of professors from the sophomore level at one school, I found that what they meant by "integration" was that Nursing of Children, the Family, and the Individual were all taught in the same quarter; however, I couldn't find any evidence of the organizing component for the integration. The group also professed to getting together to work as a team *only* to prepare assignments and exams. They candidly admitted that they felt the concept afforded them more free time to work on other projects (because they weren't in class every lecture day), but that meeting regularly to coordinate classroom activities infringed on their academic freedom and took too much time. They stated that the arrangement had been established based on their individual academic needs.

After much reflection on the interviewing process, I narrowed my options down to two schools. One of my choices was a program in a small four-year liberal arts college that is close to home; the position was a tenure-track appointment in which I would teach Adult Health in a curriculum that was essentially built on a medical model. The other option was a private university that was a 45-minute commute from home; the position was a nontenure-track position, in which I would be teaching Health Maintenance to sophomore-level students in a curriculum that is clearly based on a nursing model.

My first choice optimally was the university, but I had to admit that I was scared to death of the position because of my lack of experience, the self-imposed mandate to work on my doctorate, the commuting time, and last, but certainly not least, the desire to maintain my family roles of wife and mother. The decision would have been so much easier if I did not need to consider my family: I would have enjoyed taking the opportunity to relocate, pursue the doctorate, and "prove" myself in the atmosphere of scholars. Given my situation and the need to fulfill all of my other roles, however, the decision became much more complicated.

The decision to teach in a small liberal arts college with a baccalaureate program seems to be the right one for me, at least for the present time. The associate degree programs and the diploma schools offered very different opportunities, as did the university setting; however, for now, I'm glad I chose to come here.

I have some questions and observations I need to share with you. I'm having a difficult time understanding the chain of command here. In the service setting the lines of authority seemed so much clearer; indeed, on the very first day everyone was handed the organizational flow chart. When you arrived, you clearly knew who your boss was. But in academe, it doesn't seem as clear, and I need some help in sorting this system out.

Within this department there is a chairperson, a curriculum coordinator, and a level leader. In the college there is a division dean, an academic dean (also titled the dean of faculty) and, of course, the president.

My confusion stems from a comment made at one of the earliest college faculty organization meetings in which a professor from another division stated that his contract did not stipulate the need to "clear things" through his department chairperson (who he obviously did not like). He stated that his employer is the college and, therefore, his immediate superior in the chain of command was the dean of faculty. Of course I got confused. I had been used to clinical teaching in a community college where the whole issue of authority lines seemed much clearer. And in that setting, the president of the union was always available to give me the information I needed about who I needed to talk to when something needed to be done if I could not find it out from the faculty handbook.

When I approached the "old timers" in my department (wouldn't they love being called that!) for their guidance, there were very different answers regarding the correct lines to follow. The first one told me, "I never do anything without clearing it through the level leader, curriculum coordinator, and the chairperson of the department." The second one told me that, "You always go to the dean of faculty." The third one offered that, "You don't get anything unless you go through Dolores." (Dolores is one of the oldest members of the department who seems to have her own contraband connection for everything from paper clips to information on tenure approvals! I'm not sure how she feels about me yet, but the other faculty members say that if she doesn't like you, you may as well not unpack your cartons of books because you won't be here long enough for them to collect dust. We'll see!) My fourth source told me that "You just ask the secretary for what you want and don't clear it with anyone." (The secretary, I'm told, has been given specific instructions that she works for the faculty. In exploring this a little further, I found out that the secretary believes they are *the* professors, giving them some kind of sovereign rights.)

My teaching partner, who is relatively new here, tells me that it really doesn't matter who you ask for things because the college views the nursing department as a necessary liability in this liberal arts college. This means that the nursing department gets the essentials that it needs to operate, and beyond that there is little else. I'm not sure I agree completely, but after only six weeks I know that I do not have a handle on the situation. I do know that our offices are small cubicles in the basement with no windows, whereas many of the other departments' faculties are above ground. Do you think this means anything?

Another question I have regarding the lines of authority is where do the NLN, the State Board, and the regional accrediting agency fit into the picture? For instance, if the NLN recommends the purchase of computer technology, can the college be "strong armed" into allocating the monies to the department for the purchase of this equipment?

Along these same lines, how does the nursing department relate to other departments on campus? I'm not sure if there is a hierarchy among departments and the faculty in them. I *do* know that tenured faculty have some rights that are different from those of nontenured faculty and faculty who are not on tenure track lines. But exactly how it all fits together is unclear to me.

My last concern for the day (I'm sure that is not true!) is whether I should consider the chairperson an enemy. Some of the older faculty in this department make comments that make me wonder whether the chairperson is a friend or foe. It is very hard to decide who to believe and who to trust. I need some good solid advice on how to negotiate this system.

DEAR HELEN:

Ah, the trials and tribulations of job hunting! Take heart—it'll be easier next time and the time after that. . . .

Your idea of using networks at professional meetings was a good way to begin to "get a feel" for what positions were available and what those schools were like (although you know you need to assess this latter point for yourself!). For future reference, other good sources of positions available in nursing education are the *Journal of Nursing Education*, *Nursing Outlook*, the *Chronicle of Higher Education*, *Nursing Research*, and *The American Nurse*. There also is nothing wrong with just writing to the dean or chairperson at a school expressing your interest in a position and sending a curriculum vitae, or CV.

Isn't it funny how we are on the same "wave length" so often? Your letter about your job search, the chain of command, and inter- and intradepartmental relations arrived just when I was experiencing confusion about the myriad relationships we encounter. I'm sure I don't have all the answers, but I can say that your questions relative to some of these issues were excellent ones. They helped me get a better handle on my own situation and deal with it effectively—I hope! I won't go into the details of my situation—I'll save that for when we have a chance to talk—but it did help me clarify some things and come to some conclusions. Maybe if I share those with you, it'll help.

I must say I particularly enjoyed your comment about how clear the lines of authority are in the service setting and how "fuzzy" they are in education. A few years ago I would have agreed with you unquestionably, but as I spend more time in the academic world, I'm not so sure.

There *are* very clear lines of communication and command in academe, and it *is* a bureaucracy. What seems different from service, though, is the emphasis placed on this and the rigidity of the hierarchy.

In education, you are told only vaguely who to go to with questions and problems. Then you're on your own to figure it out in specific situations. My guess is that your faculty handbook contains some type of organizational chart. (If it's not in your college handbook, look in your NLN Self-Study report. . . . I know it'll be in there.) But the thing that makes some of this "muddy" is that in education, the people who are involved in the delivery of the service (i.e., those responsible for the teaching and evaluation of students) are professional peers, which is not the case in service.

All academicians are minimally prepared at the master's level, and most hold the doctor's degree (even in nursing, we now have more doctorally prepared faculty). They are actively involved in research, writing, and professional organizational activities. Additionally, by the very nature of a collegiate setting, they are responsible for the students' educational experiences. You are dealing, therefore, with a group of people who are highly educated, articulate, well experienced, and recognized experts in their fields. Clearly, they are not going to be pigeon holed and just "take it" when someone says, "You're only allowed to speak to your department chair." In contrast, when a staff nurse presents a proposal to her head nurse that is unacceptable, she may just let it drop. A faculty member probably won't.

I sit on a number of university committees with the academic vice president and the deans of various schools and colleges on campus. Even though I'm a faculty member without administrative responsibility, I call the deans by their first name, and we talk like colleagues. This is especially true with my own dean! Although the dean is my "boss" organizationally, she also is my colleague professionally. I don't think this is typically true in the service setting, and I think it contributes to some of the confusion about lines of authority in academe.

The faculty member you mentioned from the other department was right. The fact is that, similar to the service setting, individuals are employed technically by the institution, not by the department. However, he is dead wrong in following that logic through to conclude that his immediate superior in the chain of command is the dean of faculty! His immediate supervisor—and yours—is the department chairperson.

When a faculty member has a request, a problem, or a proposal, it should be presented to the department chairperson. If the chairperson refuses the request or proposal or opts not to help with the problem, and the faculty member believes the decision is unjust, then it should be pursued at the next level. In your case, this would be the dean of faculty. Of course, the chairperson should be kept informed of any such further action. (In my situation, because we are organized differently, I would go to the assistant dean for undergraduate nursing studies and then to the dean of the College of Nursing.)

When faculty bypass the "chain of command" in any institution, the same results often occur: anger, frustration, mistrust, miscommunication, etc. When faculty are *allowed* to do so (i.e., when the dean of faculty listens to the faculty member and takes action without involving the chairperson), it undermines the system and dilutes the chairperson's power and ability to do the job. In my opinion, that is far from a desirable situation.

In nursing departments, matters tend to be complicated by having curriculum coordinators, and level or course leader positions. As I have experienced such positions, they have been purely managerial or coordinating ones and nothing more. Technically, then, those people usually have no official power or administrative responsibility. It would seem to me that if your department has such positions, they should be depicted on your organizational chart, and there should be a written position description for each. If this isn't the case, maybe you need to ask your department chairperson to address the question.

Generally, a faculty member's day-to-day interactions would be with the level leader (or course leader). Questions about course content, student evaluation forms, classroom assignments, teaching support material, and so on usually can be answered by the level or course leader. The level leader, however, has no more right to dictate the details of the course than does the department chairperson. Such decisions are made either by the individual faculty member teaching the course (I won't go into my academic freedom harangue now!) or by the faculty group approved to make curriculum decisions. Remember, the curriculum is the responsibility of the entire faculty.

To get back to your letter . . . I had to smile when I read about the different answers you got from the "old timers." Smile, because it's so typical . . . and so real.

Because of the emphasis on scholarliness in a university, people tend to think that faculty members are different from everyone else and somehow don't get caught up in acting in petty ways, politicking, and playing the system. Of course, you know as well as I do that just is not true. All those things go on just like they do in other institutions and with other groups. People form alliances, they make decisions differently, and they interpret procedures in uniquely individual ways.

Given the various ways in which people interpret procedures, you can see how one old timer—who once was the level leader or curriculum coordinator, who enjoyed some power in that position, and who now has her best friend in that position—will tell you everything must be cleared through the curriculum coordinator. On the other hand, the old timer who once had a problem which the chairperson couldn't resolve but the dean of faculty could, will tell you to go through the dean. Finally, some individual faculty members have developed such a power base over the years that they *are* the ones who "pull all the strings" on a number of matters and the ones to go to with a request or problem.

It all gets so complicated I can't begin to sort out all the possibilities. Let me just say that politics operates in the university just as it does anywhere else. Anyone who wants to survive and flourish in a particular group has to learn what the norms of that group are and how to play the political game . . . at least to some extent. (Some systems are so political that you use up all your energy trying to anticipate who will do what and how others will react that you have no energy left to teach and do all the other things you need to do! To me, it's not worth it to stay in that kind of system, and I would seriously consider leaving.) There *are* proper lines of authority, there *should be* position descriptions to clarify roles and responsibilities, and the faculty and chairperson *should* remember they are there because of the students, and that's what they should worry about the most. We are all in this together, and wouldn't we be able to move so much farther if we didn't waste so much time fighting each other? Oh well.

I don't know how much more I can say or what advice I can give you. This whole aspect of university life can be very frustrating, but somehow I find some comfort in knowing we're no different from most other groups and systems.

The situations you described are confusing and do make you wonder what sense can be made of it all. In thinking about how to manage these situations, though, remember that you have no difficulty working cooperatively with others. Your commitment to providing your students with quality learning experiences is clear. Additionally, you are not out to seek power purely for the sake of power. I trust you'll make the best decisions in some of these crazy situations. Let me know how it continues to go.

1

The First Faculty Appointment

Entering any new workplace can be an exciting and challenging experience, but becoming a nurse educator for the first time offers particular opportunities. Nurse educators have the potential to affect the nation's health because the students they teach will have the responsibility of providing care to large segments of the population, a point that may not have occurred to the beginning nurse educator. Recognition of this fact may be both stimulating and frightening. To prepare for this responsibility, particular information will be essential.

EDUCATIONAL PREPARATION

In assuming the role of nurse educator and carrying out the responsibilities inherent in it, a certain degree of prerequisite knowledge is essential. A combination of clinical abilities and educational theory provides the strongest base from which to enter the teaching arena and enhances one's ability to perform. Educated solely as a clinical practitioner or solely as an educator limits one's abilities to function most effectively and efficiently in this role that integrates teaching and evaluation.

Locasto and Kochanek (1989) assert that the transition from graduate student to nurse educator is very similar to the reality shock phenomenon reported by Kramer (1974). New nurse educators, like new graduates, experience the stages of reality shock: honeymoon phase, shock and rejection phase, recovery and resolution phase. All of the stages ultimately lead to the acquisition of a realistic perspective on the new role. The new nurse educator can expect "highs and lows" related to the new experience. The best way to facilitate the transition is to collect as much information as possible before entering the position. Assessing one's skills as both clinical practitioner and educator will provide much of the factual data needed to make decisions related to career goals.

MAPPING ONE'S CAREER

During the early stages of development as a bedside nurse, individuals can recall hearing nursing faculty speak repeatedly about the need to be goal directed in the care of patients. To optimize care of one's career in the academic system, it is equally important to be goal directed. The new nurse educator should identify career goals early. Defining both short- and long-term career goals is essential. To realize particular goals, it will be necessary to gather as much data about the potential position as possible to make decisions.

The questions that need to be asked are not unlike those raised in obtaining the first nursing staff position: In what geographic area do I need or wish to live? In which type of nursing program do I prefer to work? What sort of benefits do I need and want? In what clinical areas to I feel most comfortable? What salary do I need or want? What is my philosophy of nursing education? Am I willing to take a position for a short term and move to another institution at a later time? What is the maximum amount of distance I want to commute? And are there other prerequisites for employment? All of these questions will need answering before beginning to look for a position.

In answering the questions identified, the new nurse educator will be able to focus the search for a position. For instance, if an individual is master's prepared and identifies a doctor's degree as a long-term goal, it is important to find a position in a school of nursing that will financially support these activities or at least will place less demands in the areas of service and scholarship while one meets that goal. If a long-term goal is to teach in a graduate program, a new nurse educator may wish to locate a school of nursing that houses an undergraduate and graduate program, and supports faculty teaching in both.

Only the persons pursuing particular positions can decide what their personal long- and short-term goals are and what are the best ways to reach those goals. Once a decision is made about what is most important, the nurse educator can begin to look for the desired position in a suitable geographic area.

LOCATING THE FIRST POSITION

When the questions listed earlier have been answered and long- and short-terms goals are developed, the nurse educator can begin to select potential schools of nursing at which to interview. Several sources are available for locating positions. Some of the ones offered may differ from those used to obtain the first nursing practice position.

One of the most useful ways of locating a potential employment setting is to use informal networks. Ask around, talk to colleagues. Valuable information can be collected this way. Frequently individuals who have worked in a particular program or have friends who have worked in it will be good sources of data. Be cautious when negative information is shared about a school of nursing, however, and remember that such views are very personal in nature and may not be viewed similarly by the applicant. If the program is appealing, pursue it further and try to "tease out" the sources of major criticisms. If negative statements are made repeatedly about the program, the nurse educator still has the option to interview and draw conclusions based on what is seen and heard at the time of the interview. The other option is to terminate the inquiry based on what has been offered. Similarly, if everything heard about an institution is wonderful, be equally cautious. No college or university is nirvana; all will have their own weaknesses as well as strengths. It will be the job of the person interested in the program to sort out what is liked, what is needed, and what can be accepted or tolerated.

In addition to using informal networks, the new teacher can also find positions listed in local newspaper advertisements; professional periodicals such as the *Journal of Nursing Education*, and *Nurse Educator*; professional newspapers such as the *American Nurse* or the *Chronicle of Higher Education*; and on bulletin boards in colleges and universities or at conventions. A job search service may be another option, but this is more useful in locating nursing service or educational administration positions rather than in entry faculty positions.

Other sources of information about potential employing institutions include college catalogs, former students, and members of organizations that have affiliations with the school, such as hospitals or other clinical agencies. Although these sources may be biased, they will provide valuable data about the school of nursing and the college or university in which it is located that will assist in making the final decision.

To make a formal application, write a letter to the school. Nowak and Grindel (1984) describe how to write a letter and develop a résumé. This book can be a useful source of information when putting together the data that will be submitted to the prospective employer. The application letter that is written for a nurse educator position should speak to one's goals relative to the teaching role and, if possible, should demonstrate some knowledge of the program. Depending on the structure of the institution, the letter is directed to the administrative director of the program, the chairperson of the search committee, or the college or university personnel department. It is very important to identify the correct person to whom the letter should be sent.

INTERVIEWING

Comparable to applying for a staff nurse position, a representative from the school of nursing usually will write or call to let the candidate know the letter of interest and résumé or curriculum vitae were received. During this communication, the representative from the program will arrange an interview appointment or will let the applicant know that his or her expertise does not meet the current needs of the school or department. Most advertised positions receive many inquiries. Being contacted for an interview acknowledges that the candidate's skill and expertise are seen as possible assets to the program.

As stated earlier, be sure to keep long- and short-term goals in mind when deciding whether to interview and during the interviewing process. If additional information is collected before the interview that leads the applicant to believe that the program would not meet career goals, then the candidate should tell the person who made the contact that he or she will not be coming for an interview. If the applicant believes that the school has the right elements to help in moving toward career goals, however, then the interview should be pursued.

When one is called to set up the interview, be sure to ask to speak to individuals who will be able to help in making a decision; such individuals might include the chairperson of the department, curriculum coordinator, or course leader. Also ask that a copy of the catalog, nursing philosophy, organizational framework, and schedule for the interview day be sent prior to the interview. By reading over this material before the interview, the candidate can begin to formulate questions and identify who the key players are within the organization. Brink (1988) suggests that the following always be kept in mind as one proceeds through the job search process:

> Your prime requirement as an individual is to do the things that will enhance your career. Consequently, when you take your first job, find out what you have to do to fulfill the requirements of your job and whether or not those requirements meet your career goals. The activities may or may not be one and the same. Whereas you may have many people monitoring your job, no one except you will monitor your career. (p. 5)

With the preceding statement in mind, be ready to ask the questions that will need to be answered to make the best choice for personal career goals. The individual starting a new career takes on more than a job.

When the interview date arrives use the same approach employed when securing the first job: dress appropriately, arrive on time or a little early, and attend to listening as much as talking. These three simple guides will go a long way in the interview process.

Before the day of the interview, the candidate should try to identify who the persons are who will conduct the formal sessions. Knowing who the people are and the positions they hold will help direct questions to the appropriate individuals. Often when the neophyte nurse educator pursues the first job there is a distinct feeling of being at the mercy of the prospective institution. Although there is a benefit to being eager for a position, remember the ultimate decision to work in a particular organization rests with the candidate. Only the applicant can decide if there is a good match.

Because teaching is a new area of opportunity for the applicant, it will be important to develop questions related to the new role. The following list offers suggestions of questions related to the various faculty expectations that should be addressed during an interview.

Teaching

1. What will my teaching assignment be?
2. How many hours of clinical teaching am I expected to do?
3. How many hours of classroom teaching are expected?
4. Would I be expected to teach outside my area of specialty?
5. What teaching strategies are typically used in the classroom?
6. How responsive are students and faculty to creative approaches to teaching?

Advising

1. How many students am I responsible for advising?
2. Will I be advising undergraduate and graduate students?
3. Will I have any responsibility for advising graduate research projects?
4. What is the role of the adviser?
5. How do students typically view advisers?

Institutional Policies and Structure

1. Is there a tenure policy? If so, what is it?
2. What is the promotion policy?
3. What exactly is the job description?
4. To whom do I report?
5. What is the length of the contract? How often is it renegotiated?
6. What is the salary?
7. What is included in the benefits package?
8. Are merit raises available, and what must I do to qualify?

Research

1. What opportunities are there for research?
2. What kinds of supports are available for scholarly work, within the department or college, or university?

Service

1. What kinds of committee responsibilities are expected?
2. Are faculty members expected to be part of recruitment activities? What is the time requirement?
3. What other expectations are there for the position?

Additional questions may be asked about the program's philosophy and how it is implemented. Similarly, the candidate may want to ask questions about the particular institution's teaching philosophy. Questions should be asked about the strategies used for teaching. Is team teaching used? Is classroom enrollment limited? What is a typical class size? Also, inquiry should be made regarding faculty practice. Are faculty members required to engage in clinical practice in addition to their teaching role? If clinical practice is expected, how is it facilitated?

These questions are offered as guides. Obviously based on the type of institution chosen, some of the questions suggested would not be pertinent. For example, applicants to junior college positions may want to focus more on teaching, advising, and service, and less on scholarship and research. The applicant will need to decide what needs to be known and collect as much information during the interview as possible.

In addition to the preceding list of suggested questions, it will be useful to find out what the institution values and what it rewards in order to establish priorities and set reasonable and meaningful time commitments (Copp, 1987). Finding the answer to the question of values and rewards may not be easy. This type of inquiry creates a situation in which carefully listening to the responses offered by those with whom the applicant interviews will be invaluable. The informality of a luncheon interview often reduces some of the rhetoric. Listening carefully should help the applicant determine the institution's real values.

In addition to the questions asked by the candidate during the interview, astute interviewers will ask questions of their own. One of the questions that might be anticipated and prepared for is what one believes he or she will be able to contribute to the institution. In today's marketplace, employers are not only interested in filling faculty positions but also in what the prospective faculty member has to contribute to the school. Colleges and universities have been under tremendous scrutiny in recent years to document that what they say they provide is being provided. Schools are also being asked to provide evidence that what students or their parents are paying for is worth it. This is one of the reasons why the candidate's perception of his or her potential contribution to the college or university may be questioned.

Another question that might be anticipated is what the candidate's plans and goals are, and how working within the particular nursing program will help meet them. Also be ready to discuss personal strengths and accomplishments to date as well as beliefs about teaching.

DECISION MAKING: WHICH POSITION IS RIGHT?

After the interview process, additional data may still need to be collected to make the best choice. First, candidates must decide which nursing program offers the opportunities most congruent with their personal short- and long-term goals. Narrowing the choices down to two or three will facilitate decision making.

Once the neophyte educator has decided on two or three schools at most, there are some other considerations to make. One of these is where is the program physically housed? Is the nursing department or college the last building on campus? What is the appearance of the physical plant in relation to other areas viewed on campus? Are faculty members sharing offices in the nursing department, whereas liberal arts faculty members have private offices? In the organizational structure does the administrative person in nursing have an equal place with respect to all of the other deans or department chairpersons?

What types of institution are the ones being considered: liberal arts colleges, full-service universities, academic health centers, junior colleges? Is the institution public or private? Is there a religious affiliation? Does the institution offer tenure? If not, is a nontenured position acceptable? What kind of reputation does the institution have? How is the clinical practice of the graduates viewed within the local health care systems?

How many faculty are employed in the department or college of nursing? How does this number compare with other departments within the institution? What is the faculty:student ratio?

In addition to asking these questions, there is a need to assess the particulars of the position. If practice and research are high priorities, is time available within the prescribed work load to fulfill this requirement? Langemo (1988) found that the average nursing faculty member works 57.5 hours per week. To reduce the stress related to the tremendous demands on faculty time, the participants in her study stated that the three most important factors to prevent burnout were reasonable work load and expectations, support and respect from administration, and recognition of teaching excellence. These three parameters can be used as indicators of a potential fit between the prospective teacher and the institution to which one is applying.

In addition to the requirements for teaching, advising, research and practice, is there an expectation that one complete the doctorate? If so, is there financial and administrative support for this activity? It is essential to determine exactly how the requirements for promotion will be managed if the new educator is required to pursue a doctoral degree. It is extremely difficult to fulfill all the expectations required in university settings and carry out doctoral study at the same time. It may be necessary to forgo promotion and merit increases until completion of the doctoral course of study.

What are the promotion practices of the institution? Are the policies consistently applied throughout the institution? de Tornyay (1988) suggests that several alternatives for promotion and tenure should be available to faculty. The long-standing tradition of published research being the major criterion for promotion is limiting. What does the institution being applied to use as the standard for promotion in rank?

A salary proposal may be offered during the interview. If so, the applicant may want to determine whether or not the offer is within the range for that rank within the particular geographic area. The way to get the most objective information regarding salary is to use salary ranges published by several sources. These include *The Chronicle of Higher Education*, the American Association of University Professors, the American Association of Colleges of Nursing, and the National League for Nursing. *The Chronicle of Higher Education* and *Academe*, the official publication of the American Association of University Professors specifically publish salary scales by rank for most institutions of higher education once a year. These two sources list average salaries of all faculty employees in the institutions, reporting by rank. This information can be an invaluable tool during salary negotiations.

Once all of the data are gathered it will be possible to sit down with career goals and analyze what is being offered and how it will best fulfill one's need. Gallagher (1988) offers a Faculty Bill of Rights, which may also assist in making a final decision. Contemplate each statement and assess it in relation to all the data collected including the observations made and the feelings experienced.

FACULTY BILL OF RIGHTS

1. Recognition of their own personhood.
2. Own and express their own feelings.
3. Have equal consideration given to suggestions.
4. Be provided with growth-producing direction.
5. Receive corrective criticism when mistakes are made.
6. Have open communication with the dean.
7. Enjoy collegiality with the dean.
8. Advocacy from the dean as (s)he interacts with university administration.
9. Work in an environment that is capable of stimulating creativity.
10. Be provided with adequate resources for performance of the faculty role. (p. 11)

Although the Faculty Bill of Rights is offered as a tool for decision making, it certainly could be used as a guide for asking questions during the interview. Remember, to be successful in taking on a new role and developing within that role one must be nurtured and valued. Neophyte nurse educators have a responsibility to themselves and to the academic community to find settings that will facilitate feelings of accomplishment and success. If this occurs it will be transmitted to students, and the whole educational setting will benefit.

When a decision is finally made about which position one will take, the nurse educator should inform the administrative director of the program or the chairperson of the search committee about the decision. Remember to also inform the appropriate individuals at the institutions not chosen. A formal thank you letter or telephone call is acceptable.

NEGOTIATING CONTRACTS

Colleges and universities ordinarily have standard types of contracts. Typically, a new faculty member receives a brief contract called a letter of appointment for the first year. This states the rank at which the individual will be hired, the length of the appointment, type of appointment (tenured or nontenured), policy and process for termination, salary, and signatures of all appropriate individuals. For instance, if the educator is being hired for an instructor position in a department of nursing within a liberal arts college, the contract may be signed by the chairperson of the department, the president of the college, and the person for whom the contract is written. The signing of the contract by all the appropriate parties generally represents a valid agreement. As a rule, specific information more fully describing various aspects of the contract are available in the faculty handbook, which also represents a legal document by which faculty and college or university administrators are bound.

After the first letter of appointment, contracts for longer periods may be available. If contracts are available for longer periods, three years is typical. In addition to knowing the terms of the contract, it is essential that the new faculty member understand the requirements of the particular rank at which one has been hired. The description of requirements of the rank will be used to direct evaluation, promotion, tenure, and salary outcomes.

Salary negotiation may need to be done before signing the contract. When this is necessary, the applicant should make the request reasonable. Rationale for the request will facilitate negotiations. The administrative officer from the nursing division will decide whether the request is reasonable in light of the rationale presented.

When deciding whether or not to accept the final offer, take into consideration that this is the first job. Outstanding performance coupled with experience will place the neophyte educator in a better position to negotiate for additional salary in time. The first position may not be the "dream position," and it probably should not be. New educators need to grow and develop and as this occurs, short- and long-term goals will change. As time goes on new challenges will be required.

SUMMARY

The process of applying for the first nurse educator position is not unlike applying for the first staff nurse position. Matching career goals with the requirements of a specific position will go a long way in providing the foundation for a flourishing career. One should set his or her sights high and work toward finding an environment that will foster personal growth and development. Recognize that all of one's personal criteria for the perfect job may not be met in the first position. As a new educator, one should select an environment that values and cultivates young scholars and that is congruent with one's goals and interests.

REFERENCES

Brink, P. B. (1988). The difference between a job and a career. *Western Journal of Nursing Research, 10*(1), 5–6.

Copp, L. A. (1987). The balancing act. *Journal of Professional Nursing, 3*(5), 265, 320.

de Tornyay, R. (1988). What constitutes scholarly activities? *Journal of Nursing Education, 27*(6), 245.

Gallagher, R. M. (1988). The role of the dean: A faculty perspective. *Nurse Educator, 13*(2), 10–11.

Kramer, M. (1974). *Reality shock: Why nurses are leaving.* St. Louis: Mosby.

Langemo, D. V. (1988). Work-related stress in baccalaureate nurse educators. *Western Journal of Nursing Research, 10*(3), 327–334.

Locasto, L. W., & Kochanek, D. (1989). Reality shock in the nurse educator. *Journal of Nursing Education, 28*(2), 79–81.

Nowak, J. B., & Grindel, C. G. (1984). *Career planning in nursing.* Philadelphia: Lippincott.

2

The Academic Unit in Nursing: Key Players and Influential Strategies

Although nursing faculty members are expected to participate fully in the affairs of the university, be professionally active and involved, and engage in scholarly activities, the largest portion of a faculty member's time, especially a relatively new faculty member, is devoted to teaching, student advisement, and committee work in one's own academic unit. It is important, therefore, that educators know their academic unit, as well as who is involved in it and how it functions, to be an integral part of it and, indeed, influence it.

FORMAL STRUCTURE

Depending on how the college or university in which the nursing program exists is organized, the academic unit in nursing may carry one of several "names": College of Nursing, School of Nursing, Division of Nursing, Nursing Department, or Nursing Program. As listed, these "names" generally denote the degree of autonomy and independence that the academic unit in nursing enjoys, from a great deal of autonomy for a college or school to more limited self-control for a program, the latter of which exists in a department of health sciences, for example.

Thus, a faculty member must know the relative standing of the nursing unit within the larger college or university system because it influences what the nursing unit can do without approval from others and who must give approval when it is necessary. Such knowledge will facilitate teachers' contributions to their programs.

Just as the academic unit may carry one of several designations, so does the head of that unit. The head of a college or school of nursing generally is known as a dean; a division may be headed by a director; a department by a chairperson; and a program by a director or head. Generally, a program director or head reports to a department chairperson who, in turn, reports to a division director or dean; the dean typically is directly responsible to the university's provost or vice-president for academic affairs. The role of the dean is discussed in more depth later in this chapter.

For the purposes of this discussion, the academic unit in nursing will be considered a college that is headed by a dean. This is the structure that provides the most autonomy for the nursing unit and usually requires additional administrative positions in it.

To accomplish the goals of a college of nursing, the dean often is assisted by several other positions. These positions might include any or all of those described subsequently.

Associate or Assistant Dean

This individual holds faculty rank and functions as the dean's "extension." The associate or assistant dean may serve as the dean's representative on university and college of nursing committees, head up special task forces in the college, write grant proposals for the college, and collaborate with faculty and other college of nursing administrators on curriculum and student affairs. Generally, this is an appointed position.

Department Chairperson or Program Director

The individual who holds this position is a faculty member who, in addition to at least some teaching responsibility, manages and provides leadership to a department (e.g., Adult Health Nursing, Psychiatric–Mental Health Nursing) or program (e.g., Graduate or Undergraduate) in the college. This person usually is responsible for course scheduling, faculty teaching assignments, faculty evaluation, clinical placements of students, student advisement, and orientation programs, as well as overall progress and evaluation of the program. As such, the chair or director usually is the "first-line" contact for a faculty member. This may be an appointed or elected position.

Level or Course Coordinator

The implementation and evaluation of the nursing curriculum may be enhanced by the designation of an individual who is intimately involved in teaching a course or a level of the program and who is responsible for coordinating the day-to-day activities of that course or level. Such activities include preparing specific material for courses, developing tests and other evaluation methods and tools, selecting textbooks, evaluating the clinical agencies used, and recommending changes needed in the course or level, all in collaboration with faculty. This may be an appointed or elected position.

Curriculum Coordinator

In some academic units, an individual is appointed or elected to coordinate all activities related to the curriculum, such as implementation of the conceptual framework and level or program objectives, implementation of curriculum changes approved by faculty, and evaluation of the curriculum. If such a position exists, it is important that the specific responsibilities of this individual be distinguished from those of the level or course coordinator, or the department chairperson or program director.

Assistant to Dean or Administrative Assistant

This individual, who may or may not hold faculty rank, often has responsibility for the administrative "details" of the college: classroom scheduling, budget preparation and monitoring, supervision of the secretarial and other college of nursing staff, and preparation of selected reports. This is an appointed position.

Thus, the formal structure of an academic unit in nursing can take many forms and involve "players" with varied titles and areas of responsibility. To be most effective in their own systems, faculty members must know these structures and areas of responsibility, and use them appropriately and effectively.

INFORMAL STRUCTURE

In addition to its formal structure, it is important that faculty members understand the informal structure within the academic unit. This is the structure one learns from a mentor or from watching and listening carefully to which issues are addressed, how decisions are made, who the powerful individuals on the faculty are, how certain faculty members influence others, and what kinds of coalitions are formed.

As is true in any other group, the informal structure of an academic unit in nursing and, indeed, of the entire university system, may be more powerful than the formal structure in facilitating or blocking change. A faculty member may get caught up in those power struggles. Thus, one must be aware of their existence, know how to use them effectively, and be cautious not to be abused by them.

For example, if faculty members wanted to propose a curriculum change, they could, in most instances, take that proposal directly to the curriculum committee. The informal system, however, may be such that the chance of seeing this proposal accepted would be enhanced if the faculty members sought out the advice of the curriculum committee chair and obtained the support of the course or level coordinator and faculty colleagues before submitting it to the committee. By knowing their allies and potential adversaries in advance, and by effectively using the informal network, faculty members are more likely to accomplish their own goals.

ROLE OF THE DEAN

Perhaps one of the "players" in the academic unit with whom nursing faculty members interact a great deal but about whom they know the least is the dean. Indeed, a recent issue of the *Chronicle of Higher Education* addressed this point through an article entitled "An Old Academic Question Revived: 'What Does a Dean Do?'" (Gold, 1988).

For years, the relationship between faculty and deans has been an unclear one. Indeed, as Freedman (1987) expressed, "at most academic institutions today, administrators seem to regard faculty members as natural enemies, if not inferiors, rather than as colleagues in a common enterprise" (p. 28). He went on to say that faculty also harbor similar feelings, and the result is a flourishing "mutual disrespect" (p. 28).

Tucker and Bryan (1987), in their analysis of the academic dean, addressed the problems and pressures with which administrators are confronted including those resulting from relationships with faculty. This idea also was supported by Bennis (1976) who asserted that an "unconscious conspiracy" exists, that faculty is a part of the conspiracy, and that this conspiracy interferes with an academic leader's ability to lead.

Writings about faculty work load, faculty burnout, and faculty morale (Austin & Gamson, 1983; Charron, 1985; Eisenhauer, 1984; Ezell, 1983) alluded to the role of administrators in creating such tensions. Much concern has been expressed about the legitimate (though not always realized) role of faculty in university governance.

All of this would seem to lead one to conclude that faculty and administrators are sworn enemies, and that only in the most unusual of circumstances would they join forces. Such an attitude does little to enhance academic programs, promote the personal and professional development of faculty, or help the institution meet its goals and fulfill its mission, nor does it recognize the mutual respect and cooperation that frequently exists among faculty and administrators.

Although it is true that faculty and administrators hold different perspectives on many academic issues, they should share the same long-range goals and be willing to collaborate in finding creative approaches to meet those goals. We teach and expect our students to be open-minded, to listen to others' viewpoints, to be sensitive to the constraints under which other people function and make decisions, and to move toward changing a system by employing valid change strategies. Perhaps those of us who teach in and administer academic programs could learn a great deal from our own advice.

As nurse clinicians, we know that when people do not understand other people's roles or what is happening around them, they often become angry and defensive. The same is true with faculty members. If they fail to understand the role of the dean and the constraints under which deans operate, they may contribute to the adversarial relationship described previously.

What *does* a dean do? In many respects, the dean's role is as complex and multidimensional as that of faculty members, although the specific aspects of the role are quite different. Indeed, Armiger (1976) spoke of the "kaleidoscopic quality of the dean's function" (p. 165).

In most institutions the dean holds an academic rank and is expected to carry some teaching assignment, albeit minimal. As an integral part of the university's and the nursing school or college's decision-making bodies, the dean may be a member of and actively participate in committees and task forces.

As a scholar, the dean is expected to continue research activities, publish, and present ideas at professional conferences. As a professional, it also is expected that the dean will maintain active involvement in appropriate professional organizations.

In addition to fulfilling these responsibilities, which are similar to those for faculty, the dean has many more dimensions to the position. The dean must be a politician—within the nursing school or college, within the university, and outside the university. Hart (1977) asserted that the dean's "most important contribution is to achieve and maintain a delicate balance between humanism, professionalism, and legalism" (p. 708). By humanism, Hart (1977) meant "a sensitive, respectful, and humane view of all the human beings she encounters" (p. 708); by professionalism, she meant "ensuring the quality of [the] program, translating professional standards into a visible reality, and . . . improving the quality and quantity of professional nursing care available to consumers" (p. 708); and by legalism, she meant "compliance with all federal, state, and local legislation" (p. 708). This balance is quite delicate and calls for many political skills.

As the person who is responsible for providing "the environment with the resources for teaching, research, and community service" (Chamings & Brown, 1984, p. 91), the dean must constantly call upon a variety of skills. To create an atmosphere of candor, openness, and trust where faculty, students, staff, and administrators work in harmony to accomplish common goals is no small task.

Oftentimes, however, these internal activities are the easier part of a dean's role. The dean is the person who must seek outside funding to maintain or advance the program, negotiate with other institutions for innovative projects, communicate with the public and with accrediting or approval bodies, and ensure the visibility and viability of the program in the larger professional community. These activities may, of necessity, take the dean away from the specific program. In a study of perceived management functions of deans of social science departments, physical science departments, and medical schools, Neumann and Neumann (1983) found that in all schools, deans were perceived as paying utmost attention to external activities, and least attention to internal activities. Faculty members who hold such perceptions may have experienced deans who were irresponsible and, indeed, did forgo involvement in the school's functioning in favor of external activities. Such perceptions, however, may also be related to the lack of understanding by faculty of this element of the dean's role.

The dean also acts as finance officer. In this role, it is the dean's responsibility to convince the university administration of the program's needs to secure adequate funds to hire qualified faculty, purchase audiovisual and computer hardware and software, support faculty attendance at professional meetings, provide for release time for faculty to write grants or conduct research, and support innovative teaching approaches. In times of increasing demands for cost containment, the dean cannot always be successful in securing all the desired funds, despite the convincing nature of the arguments presented. Unfortunately, faculty often sees the "bottom line"—namely the limited funds available—as a lack of effort on the part of the dean to secure those funds.

Even when a substantial budget for the program has been approved, the dean's position is still a precarious one. It is rare that there would be enough money in even a healthy budget to buy a personal computer for every faculty member, totally redesign and redecorate faculty offices, send all faculty members to every professional conference they might want to attend, or have a classroom ratio not in excess of 1 to 12. The dean must make some difficult decisions regarding budget expenditures, the outcome of which is that some faculty, naturally, will be unhappy. The dean, as "bearer of the bad news, [is] often blamed and seen as [a] poor manager as the need for reallocation of resources becomes more pressing" (Barritt, 1986, p. 40). As a result, the dean is in a vulnerable position.

Faculty members sometimes have a narrow view of what is im-

portant and what should take priority. They tend to think their particular request, their course, their office, or their program is of para-
mount importance and deserves the utmost attention. Indeed, at
times this is the case. But many times such requests, when compared
with those of other faculty or other programs, are not critical. When
the faculty in one old building is literally becoming ill because of poor
air circulation, the installation of new heating and cooling systems
(which may seem like a luxury to faculty who do not see the "bigger
picture") is more critical than buying another group of faculty the
newest, most sophisticated piece of laboratory equipment when what
they now have is adequate. It is the dean who has and must maintain
this broader perspective on the university's needs, directions, and
priorities.

Inherent in the dean's role is the ability to identify conflict
sources and manage conflict situations (Woodtli, 1987). Indeed, managing conflict is, no doubt, an element of the dean's role on a daily basis. The dean often becomes involved in conflict at many levels: faculty and administration, students and administration, faculty and
faculty, faculty and student, and so on. In most instances, faculty-fac-
ulty and faculty-student conflicts are brought to the dean only if they
have not been resolved elsewhere. The dean then assumes the role of
final "judge" and arbiter. If an angry student, an angry parent, or an
irate faculty member bypasses the normal "channels of communication" in the institution and goes directly to a vice-president or to the
president, however, it is the dean who is called to explain the situation
and see to its resolution. The management of such situations calls for
a dean who is astute, sensitive, quick thinking, and "in touch" with
what is going on in the school or college.

The conflicts for deans do not arise entirely from external situations, however. Many times conflicts arise from the clashing of the
dean's past experience in a faculty role and sympathy toward faculty's
positions on an issue with the need to be concerned about the good of
the university as a whole and to be an administrative "team player."
Austin and Gamson (1983) have analyzed this seemingly dichotomous
individual and concluded that intrapersonal conflicts may be abun-
dant for the dean who has one foot in administration and one foot in
academics. Such personal conflicts can be most difficult for deans
when the two constituencies they represent—faculty and administra-

tors—are at odds with each other. Added to this is the fact that the dean is relatively isolated from the rest of the faculty group.

To whom does the dean go with a problem or a concern? Faculty can go to one another or to their level coordinator or to the dean. The dean can go to dean colleagues or to the vice-president with some matters, but the expectation generally is that such interactions will be minimal. In other words, the dean is expected to be capable of handling problems. Additionally, if the problem is discipline specific, there typically is no one else in the university at or above the dean's level with whom to discuss the matter. This relative isolation has been addressed by several authors (Austin & Gamson, 1983; Chamings & Brown, 1984; Torres, 1981), and it can have serious outcomes.

Partridge (1983) concluded that the dean's role is both prestigious and contemptuous as a result of having to serve as a bridge between faculty and the university's top administration. Torres (1981) asserted that deans are vulnerable as a result of being primarily accountable to students and to the health care consumer. Woolley (1981) implied that the dean must repeatedly defend why nursing belongs in the university and why it needs the resources it does as a result of the less-than-positive image of nursing held by non-nursing faculty and many administrators in a university. Thus, the role is not an easy one.

Although written a number of years ago, Armiger's (1976) characterization of what a dean needs to be is just as relevant today as it was then. The dean of today needs to be resilient, welcome participatory governance, be willing to achieve goals through the faculty, and value openness and being available to students and faculty. More important, however, Armiger (1976) described the dean of the future: a statesperson, a leader in health care as well as in education, an advocate for increased interdisciplinary exchange and cooperation, a consumer of computerized management systems to facilitate decision making, a community activist, and a futurist.

UNIQUE CONCERNS OF DEAN OF NURSING

In addition to fulfilling these expectations, which are common to deans of a variety of schools or colleges, the dean of a nursing program has some very unique demands and concerns. These can complicate the role enormously, add to the stress and tension associated with the role, and affect the relationship between the dean and faculty.

All deans must be concerned about the quality of the students enrolled in their programs. They are aware that the quantity of students must be adequate if their programs are to remain vital and viable. Deans of nursing, in light of the declining enrollments recently experienced in nursing programs nationwide, also must be concerned about the actual survival of their programs.

At a time when the number of students choosing nursing programs is lower than it was in the early 1980s, deans of nursing need to argue for more university resources, not less. The dean needs to argue for the appointment of a nurse recruiter or the reduction of faculty teaching loads to allow them to pursue recruitment activities actively. The dean of nursing needs to argue for more "perks," such as better financial aid packages or guaranteed on-campus housing, to attract nursing applicants to the program. Also, the dean needs to argue to retain faculty (despite fewer students to teach) so that safe and educationally sound teacher-student ratios can be maintained in the clinical and classroom settings. Although the recruitment of students is not the dean's job alone, it is the dean who is looked to and held responsible when the nursing program does not "carry its own weight" on campus.

Deans of most professional schools (e.g., business schools) must carry the burden of meeting the standards set by accrediting bodies, and nursing is no exception. In addition, however, deans of nursing also are concerned about the constraints placed on the program by the profession's approving body (i.e., State Board of Nursing) and the pressures associated with preparing graduates for the licensing examination. These are concerns with which most other deans do not have to deal.

As a result of these external pressures, deans of nursing typically are compelled to be involved in curriculum design, implementation, and evaluation activities perhaps more so than other deans. The dean's role, authority, and responsibility for decision making related to curriculum are unclear, however, because universities generally adhere to the caveat that "the curriculum belongs to the faculty." In a study of 52 deans and 451 faculty, Higgs (1978) found that there was little agreement among faculty about the dean's precise role regarding curriculum questions, although they did agree the dean should be involved to some degree. The deans, however, expected to have and saw themselves as having greater involvement in curriculum decisions than faculty did. Thus, the question of who provides curriculum leadership is one that seems particularly relevant in a discussion of the role of nursing deans.

The nursing dean faces additional unique challenges in that the position often yields the only female member of the university's "administrative team." Despite the strength, articulateness, and political savvy of an individual, a female dean may face barriers in an academic setting that is and has traditionally been male-dominated that other deans may not face. This also reinforces the isolation a nursing dean may experience (Chamings & Brown, 1984).

Nursing faculty members also are predominantly female and by comparison do not carry a long history of being actively and intimately involved in the world of academe. In addition, most nursing educators nationwide are not doctorally prepared (American Association of Colleges of Nursing, 1987, p. 7). Nursing faculty members typically are not as productive as scholars in other disciplines owing, in part, to (a) lack of doctoral preparation, (b) extensive clinical involvement, (c) heavy work loads, and (d) limited tradition as scholars. It falls on the dean of nursing to explain and defend these circumstances to peers and superiors throughout the university and, simultaneously, to continue to "push" faculty to be more comparable with other university faculty. Thus, the dean of a nursing program faces yet another unique challenge.

It is widely known that nursing academic programs are more costly than are programs in many other disciplines, and studies have been undertaken (Brown, 1982; Bryson, 1982; *Cost Estimating Models*, 1986; Starck & Williams, 1988) to determine that cost. When federal funds supporting nursing education were plentiful, not much question was raised about the expense of nursing programs. With severely limited federal funds for nursing education and with the nationwide trend toward cost consciousness and cost containment, combined with the previously mentioned reduced enrollments, deans of nursing are put on the defensive more and more frequently. Rarely does a dean of nursing attend a budget, planning, or priorities meeting without being "armed" with any number of statistics, projections, and calls for well-educated nurses. As a result of these and similar pressures for accountability, deans of nursing are, in Torres's (1981, p. 1) words, "vulnerable and oppressed."

Finally, deans of nursing programs are in a position in the university that is unlike that of their fellow deans because of the extensive relations the program has with clinical agencies in the community. If the university values these community ties, the dean's position may be enhanced. If such relations are viewed as a nuisance and one more thing that puts nursing out of synch with the rest of the university, however, the nursing program may be seen as a liability and the dean, once again, put in the position of defending the importance of these interinstitutional relationships.

In a series of monographs published by the American Association of Colleges of Nursing (*Have You Ever Thought of Being a Dean*, 1981), an analysis of the dean as administrator, scholar, colleague, and person is provided. Through this analysis, one gains an understanding of the complexities of the dean's role, the challenges facing deans of nursing now and in the future, and the qualities needed to implement the dean's role successfully.

Armiger (1976) outlined the characteristics of and qualities important in a dean as follows: the dean must be a "paragon of nursing science" (p. 167); the dean must provide for and participate in academic governance; the dean must be a curriculum expert; the dean must be skilled in finance and fund raising; and the dean must engage in future-oriented planning. Baj (1983) asserted that the dean of nursing must be knowledgeable about management and leadership theories and be able to apply those theories effectively; he or she also must be sensitive to the unique needs of the students in the program and "facilitate innovative directions from the faculty" (p. 20) to meet those unique needs.

The importance of enhancing and promoting positive relations with the university's local community and with the nursing community is a vital function of the nursing school or college dean. Indeed, "the dean is, to the outside world, that college of nursing. As chief administrator it is her task to serve as its spokesperson" (Reres, 1981, p. 48). Thus, the dean must be articulate, knowledgeable, current, and an advocate for collaborative enterprises.

The dean also must be flexible and comfortable with change, one of the most pervasive characteristics of contemporary higher education. In fact, the dean's "chances for success in meeting the formidable challenge of the future will be enhanced by a new open-mindedness, a new way of thinking about management and decision making" (Brahney, 1981, p. 2), as well as "an inquiring and receptive attitude" (p. 5).

Finally, the dean must be open with the faculty, be willing to share problems and successes, and involve the faculty in decision making related to the nursing program. The role of collaborator is one of the most important roles the dean plays; faculty members also play a similar role with one another and with the dean. In an increasingly competitive world, such collegial interaction is necessary for growth and, perhaps, for survival.

It can be seen from this analysis that the dean of a nursing program frequently is in a position to explain nursing, nursing trends, and the unique features of the nursing program. The dean also is called on frequently to defend the atypical aspects of the nursing faculty role, argue for increased resources despite being in a poor position to bargain, and manage varied and numerous conflicts on a daily basis. The dean's position is enhanced greatly when administration and faculty work collaboratively as colleagues instead of fighting each other as natural enemies.

COLLABORATION BETWEEN FACULTY AND ADMINISTRATORS

Keenan and Brown (1985) stated unequivocally that, "the time is now for accountable, responsible, participatory management that involves faculty and administrators in easing the cost-income squeeze" (p. 549). Indeed, "to ensure an organization's financial solvency, its administrators and faculty members must work cooperatively to solve problems and make decisions" (Keenan & Brown, 1985, p. 549).

The idea of faculty, deans, and other administrative personnel collaborating to achieve mutual goals is not foreign. The extent to which this idea is operationalized, however, is questionable. It would benefit both faculty and administrators if they joined forces and worked together as colleagues rather than viewing each other as foes. The dean's efforts to advance the nursing program will be enhanced greatly by faculty support; faculty tenure, promotion, and career development could be influenced significantly by a dean who takes an active role in facilitating faculty development.

It is important for faculty members to understand the multifaceted nature of an administrator's role, particularly the dean. They also must be willing to support the dean in efforts to advance the program and the profession on campus, and secure resources for the program. In addition, faculty members need to realize that student recruitment, fiscal prudence, and political savvy are not within the domain of the administrator alone. Faculty also share in these responsibilities.

Of course, faculty members are responsible for implementing the curriculum appropriately, teaching in a way consistent with the university's mission, using varied teaching strategies to enhance student learning, and pursuing their own professional development. Additionally, however, they are responsible for being a "team member" within the nursing school or college and working collaboratively with their peers, the dean, and others who hold some type of administrative responsibility.

The dean would do well to be open with faculty, involve them in decision making, and make them aware of the problems facing the nursing program. To keep such matters from the faculty contributes to mistrust, leads faculty to be concerned about empire building on the part of the dean, and underestimates the degree to which faculty want to be involved and the impact they can have.

The dean and the administrative "team" should nominate nursing faculty members for appointment to university committees as a way to increase the visibility of nursing on campus and improve nursing's image; faculty members have to be willing to accept this role, prepare well for meetings of these committees, and be articulate spokespersons for nursing. All members of the nursing unit should use their professional networks to secure opportunities for faculty members to publish, become involved in research, or hold office in professional organizations; faculty members, again, need to be willing to take advantage of such opportunities and not ignore them.

Individual faculty members should invite their respective deans or the deans' representatives to speak in classes or attend committee meetings where their expertise would be valuable. Administrators, in turn, must value these opportunities to participate in the educational program more widely and not refuse such invitations regularly. Faculty members should seek out the dean for career advisement, feedback on manuscripts or grant proposals, and advice on other professional matters; the dean has to be willing to give the appropriate input, advice, or feedback.

If the faculty and administration were to recognize and use each other's strengths to the fullest instead of focusing on each other's faults or limitations, the outcome could be a more professionally satisfied dean, a more involved and effective administrative "team," a more challenged and fulfilled faculty, and a higher quality educational program for students. The benefits of collaboration are many, and the ways to achieve it are innumerable. All that is needed is understanding, trust, mutual respect, and a willingness to take the first step.

SUMMARY

Nurse faculty members can be more effective and satisfied in their roles when they know the areas of responsibility of those with whom they interact frequently. One's particular academic unit may be composed of individuals carrying titles similar to administrative assistant, curriculum coordinator, course or level coordinator, and department chairperson, program director or dean. Although one interacts regularly with course or level coordinators, it is the dean (or department chairperson) who plays a most significant role in the system, and it is precisely this role that faculty frequently know least well.

The role of a nursing dean today is challenging and complex, and it requires a number of unique characteristics. Many of these same qualities and demands, however, also apply to associate or assistant deans, department chairpersons or program directors, level or course coordinators, and curriculum coordinators.

In offering some advice for faculty moving into or contemplating an administrative role, Beidler (1984) stated the following: "Think colleague. It is not an enemy camp. Academic administrators are not the foe" (p. 90). It would seem that everyone involved—faculty, students, parents, consumers, and the profession at large—gains from a collaborative relationship between faculty and administrators. This collaboration can be achieved more readily and outcomes influenced more effectively if faculty members know the "key players" in their own systems.

REFERENCES

American Association of Colleges of Nursing. (1987). *Faculty salary report 1986–1987*. Washington, DC: Author.

Armiger, B., Sr. (1976). The educational crisis in the preparation of deans. *Nursing Outlook, 24*(3), 164–168.

Austin, A. E., & Gamson, Z. F. (1983). *Academic workplace: New demands, heightened tensions*. Washington, DC: Association for the Study of Higher Education.

Baj, P. A. (1983). The role of the academic nursing administrator in baccalaureate programs for the registered nurse. *Nursing Leadership, 6*(1), 16–21.

Barritt, E. R. (1986). The vulnerability of deans [Sounding Board]. *Nursing Outlook, 34*(1), 40.

Beidler, P. G. (1984). Some advice for would-be administrators from a professor who's been there [Point of View]. *Chronicle of Higher Education, 28*(4), 90.

Bennis, W. (1976). *The unconscious conspiracy: Why leaders can't lead*. New York: Amacon.

Brahney, J. H. (1981). Higher education management: The name of the game is change. *Administrator's Update, 3*(1), 1–6.

Brown, E. L. (1982). *Analyzing the cost of baccalaureate nursing education — Comparing and analyzing expenditure factors in nursing education*. New York: National League for Nursing.

Bryson, J. (1982). *Cost-effective management in schools of nursing — Cost-effective management: Its implications for schools of nursing*. New York: National League for Nursing.

Chamings, P. A., & Brown, B. J. (1984). The dean as mentor. *Nursing & Health Care, 5*(2), 88–91.

Charron, S. A. (1985). Role issues and the nurse educator. *Journal of Nursing Education, 24*(2), 77–79.

Cost estimating models for baccalaureate nursing education programs. (1986). Rockville, MD: USHHS, PHS, HR&SA, BPH, DON.

Eisenhauer, L. (1984). Variables associated with perceived role conflict and role ambiguity in nursing faculty [Abstract]. *Nursing Outlook, 32*(3), 174.

Ezell, A. S. (1983). Anarchy and revolution within educational organizations of nursing. In N. L. Chaska (Ed.), *The nursing profession: A time to speak* (pp. 70–90). New York: McGraw-Hill.

Freedman, M. (1987). At most academic institutions, administrators seem to regard professors as natural enemies [Opinion]. *Chronicle of Higher Education, 33*(47), 28.

Gold, J. J. (1988). An old academic question revived: 'What does a dean do?' [Opinion]. *Chronicle of Higher Education, 34*(17), B6.

Hart, S. E. (1977). The dean is seated at her desk. *Nursing Outlook, 25*(11), 708–712.

Have you ever thought of being a dean? (1981). (Executive Development Series I: Volume I—The Dean as Administrator: Roles, Functions and Attributes; Volume II—The Dean as Person: Rights and Responsibilities; Volume III—The Dean as Colleague: Dean, Student, Faculty, Administrative Relationships; Volume IV—The Dean as Scholar: Clinical Competence, Teaching, Research and Publication). Washington, DC: American Association of Colleges of Nursing.

Higgs, Z. R. (1978). Expectations and perceptions of the curricular leadership role of administrators of nursing education units. *Nursing Research, 27*(1), 57–63.

Keenan, M. J., & Brown, E. L. (1985). Collaboration braces schools against eroding resources. *Nursing & Health Care, 6*(10), 549–551.

Neumann, L., & Neumann, Y. (1983). Faculty perceptions of deans' and department chairpersons' management functions. *Higher Education, 12*(2), 205–214.

Partridge, R. (1983). The decanal role: A dilemma of academic leadership. *Journal of Nursing Education, 22*(2), 59–61.

Reres, M. E. (1981). The dean as administrator: Roles, functions, and attributes. In *Have you ever thought of being a dean?* (pp. 44–52). Washington, DC: American Association of Colleges of Nursing.

Starck, P. L., & Williams, W. E. (1988). What does nursing education cost? Turning the question around. *Journal of Professional Nursing, 4*(1), 38–44.

Torres, G. (1981). The nursing education administrator: Accountable, vulnerable, and oppressed. *Advances in Nursing Science, 3*(3), 1–16.

Tucker, A., & Bryan, R. A. (1987). *The academic dean: Dove, dragon, diplomat?* New York: Macmillan.

Woodtli, A. O. (1987). Deans of nursing: Perceived sources of conflict and conflict-handling modes. *Journal of Nursing Education, 26*(7), 272–277.

Woolley, A. S. (1981). Nursing's image on campus. *Nursing Outlook, 29*(8), 460–466.

3

Nursing as an Integral Part of the Academic Community

One goal that nursing leaders strove to achieve with the push to move nursing education into the mainstream of higher education was to help the profession gain recognition as an academic discipline and as an integral part of any academic system. Such individuals made significant progress in helping nursing become a valuable and valued aspect of many institutions. Nursing faculty should be alert to the positioning of their programs in their colleges or universities so that this progress will not be lost, particularly as many nursing programs have shrunk in size and increased in cost.

POSITION OF NURSING IN ACADEME

The degree of influence that individuals or programs have in any organization is determined by the amount of responsibility they have, the kind of decision-making activities in which they participate, their place in the hierarchical or organizational structure, their comparability with other disciplines or programs in the organization, and their geographic location, among other factors. One cannot deny that an academic institution is a political arena. In fact, Moore (1984) noted that leadership in the academic world is as competitive and political as anywhere else and shared the following anecdote to support his claim:

Woodrow Wilson reportedly once said that he learned about politics from the faculty at Princeton and then went to Washington to practice among the amateurs. (p. 219)

Nursing faculty, then, would do well to be aware of the "politics" of the system and astutely assess where they "fit in" as well as how they can influence that system.

Hierarchical Structure

In examining the status or extent of power that nursing may have on a college or university campus, faculty should assess where their program is located in the organization's hierarchy. If nursing is a *program* in a *department* that is in a *division* that, in turn, is in a *college*, one would assume that nursing does not have much power or influence.

This type of hierarchical arrangement places a great deal of "distance" and several intermediaries between the nursing faculty or nursing program director and the individual who has ultimate responsibility for that program, namely, the dean of the college. In such instances, the dean—except if his or her background is in nursing—is not close to or especially familiar with the unique needs of nursing programs and the current issues facing the profession; it may be quite difficult, therefore, for the dean to convey those special features to the college or university vice-president for academic affairs or president when arguing for resources or projecting trends and needs for the future. As a result, nursing may not fare as well as in other structures.

When the nursing program is headed by its own dean, conversely, nursing is likely to be in a much stronger position on campus. In such situations, the nursing dean is well aware of nursing's unique needs and contributions, can address such issues more knowledgeably, and holds a position comparable with the heads of other academic disciplines, such as business, engineering, or law.

Thus, nursing faculty may wish to reflect on its position in the hierarchical structure and act to initiate some change in that structure if it does not provide for the type of representation they believe is needed. Of course, such a change will not occur simply because nursing faculty wish it to be so; they must demonstrate that change is deserved, and that it will benefit the academic institution.

Comparability with Other Disciplines

One of the ways to demonstrate that greater autonomy within the collegiate structure is warranted is for nursing faculty to be comparable with faculty in other disciplines in terms of their credentials, scholarship, and knowledge of the academic world. Although nursing's history in academe is not as long as that of many other disciplines, nursing faculty must hold themselves to the same standards used to judge faculty in those other areas.

The head of the nursing program should hold the same credentials held by other program heads (e.g., an earned doctorate), be an accomplished academic, be an articulate spokesperson for nursing, and be politically astute. He or she should know how to manage a budget, be fully aware of the trends and issues affecting the profession and nursing education, be visionary, and be able to both manage and lead the nursing faculty and nursing profession.

Nursing faculty members themselves must hold the same academic credentials as their colleagues in other disciplines, and engage in scholarly, professional, practice, or service activities as a regular part of their faculty role. In addition, they should hold themselves to the same standards for appointment, promotion, and tenure as are used for other faculty and not "make excuses" for why nursing cannot be held to the same level of expectation.

It is only through parity with their academic peers that nursing faculty will be recognized as an integral part of the academic system. Such comparability of accomplishments puts nursing faculty in a position to be respected and recognized as experts in their own right: this will do much to advance nursing within the college or university.

Participation in Decision-Making Activities

One of the criticisms frequently made of nursing faculty members is their lack of participation in college or university governance and other activities. Often cited as a major reason for this is the fact that nurse educators are off campus for large blocks of time because of clinical teaching responsibilities, and there is no doubt this is a reality with which one has to deal; however, there are ways to manage this situation.

First, nursing faculty members need to volunteer to serve on institutional committees or accept such appointments when they are offered. By constantly refusing to seek or accept such appointments, nursing faculty members convey a message that they are not interested in or willing to give their time and talent to activities that are outside their "little corner of the world." They also may lead other members of the larger academic community to question whether nursing faculty are even knowledgeable of the issues and concerns facing other disciplines and the institution as a whole.

Once they are members of committees or task forces, nursing faculty may need to assess the committees in which they are involved. Do they sit on the college or university senate or assembly, or other policy-making body? Are they members of the institutional rank and tenure committee? Do they serve on search committees for major university appointments, such as president, provost, academic vice-president, or director of research? Are they represented on task forces that deal with academic issues (e.g., a core curriculum or writing across the curriculum) and larger university concerns (e.g., university accreditation or strategic planning for the institution)? In order that their colleagues in nursing are well aware of the "big picture" of the university and in order that they have an opportunity to influence larger decisions, nursing faculty must be integral parts of these types of powerful decision-making bodies.

If nursing faculty are members of committees and task forces such as those mentioned here and they have difficulty attending meetings because of clinical teaching, advisement, and nursing department responsibilities, some action may need to be taken. Committees should be willing to rotate their meting times to accommodate the schedules of all members so that one member is not constantly unable to participate; the responsiveness of the committee to a suggestion such as this will give a clue as to how valued nursing's input is to the tasks at hand.

Another approach to deal with this problem is to reexamine the faculty member's teaching assignment during a given semester. If it is known that the major work of a particular committee (e.g., a search committee) will occur during a given time frame, the nursing department chair may, for example, structure that faculty member's time so that there is no clinical teaching, the clinical teaching is at an agency much closer to campus, no nursing committee work is expected during that time, advisees are reassigned to other faculty, or classroom teaching is scheduled for an evening section rather than during the day. In other words, if the nursing department itself values nursing's input at the university level, several options may be available to help the department achieve the level of involvement it desires.

Finally, if nursing is to be truly integral to the overall institution, faculty members must be willing to chair as well as serve on college-wide committees, task forces, and special projects. This role gives visibility to the individual and to the nursing department, demonstrates the leadership abilities which nursing faculty members have, and shows the broad perspective and multiple talents that so many nurse educators possess. When other members of the academic community see nursing faculty functioning in such leadership roles and making valuable contributions to the particular committee and the larger university, their respect for nursing increases, and the collegiality among faculty peers is enhanced.

Geographic Location

One final consideration that nursing faculty may want to make regarding the role they play in the college or university is their geographic location. Is the nursing department housed in the basement of the oldest building on the outskirts of campus? Or is it in a building comparable with other departments and located in the heart of the campus? Are nursing faculty offices cramped and poorly furnished, whereas those of other faculty groups are spacious and well appointed? Is the nursing faculty member always expected to go to someone else's "territory" for meetings? Or are meetings occasionally held in the nursing building or office area?

Such considerations may seem trivial in the larger scheme of higher education issues, but they do convey messages about the relative importance and power of various people and programs. If nursing holds a central place on campus in adequate facilities, they should strive to maintain that position and even suggest that meetings be held there, if possible. If, conversely, nursing is relegated to the basement on the far reaches of campus and is isolated from the mainstream of the institution's activities, they need to strategize on how to overcome that deficit.

NURSING'S VALUE ON CAMPUS

In addition to examining their position in the hierarchical structure, parity with academic colleagues, participation in campus-wide decision-making activities, and geographic location, nursing faculty members may also wish to reflect on other ways in which their value and expertise are recognized. This can take many forms.

Are members of the nursing faculty asked to consult with college or university representatives regarding the health services provided on campus? When some health-related issue arises, do members of the university community seek out the nursing department for advice and information? Is the institution willing to sponsor, advertise, and support the nursing department's annual health fair?

When the institution is preparing for its regional reaccreditation visit, are representatives from nursing asked to play a major role in that process, given their experience and expertise with accreditation and self-evaluation? When asked to nominate individuals for regional accreditation site visitors, does the president put forth the names of nursing faculty?

Does the research director on campus scan grant sources for funds to support the research being conducted by nursing faculty? Does the university librarian consult with the nursing faculty about new library resources and services and how they can best meet the unique needs of nursing students?

Are nursing faculty and students involved in interdisciplinary activities and programs? Do significant college or university representatives, such as the president or provost, attend and support nursing department functions (e.g., research days, special lectures, honor society inductions)?

Is the campus food service willing to open one of the cafeterias early two or three days each week so nursing students who live on campus can have breakfast and still be at their clinical agencies on time? Is the campus newspaper willing to publish an ongoing column on health-related issues, written by nursing faculty and students?

In these and many other ways, nursing faculty members can gauge if they are integral to the broader academic community or peripheral to it. The clues as to whether or not nursing is valued within the university community are varied and come from many sources.

SUMMARY

Nursing's educational leaders fought long and hard to establish nursing within institutions of higher learning, but this struggle is far from over. In fact, with reduced enrollments in nursing and an increased concern for cost in most universities, this struggle is likely to intensify.

Nursing faculty must work at being visible on, valued in, and vital to the academic community—goals that will not come without some degree of effort. In those academic institutions in which nurse educators have put forth such an effort, nursing is seen as a viable, significant part of the institution and its mission, and nursing plays an important role in all aspects of those colleges and universities. When this is achieved, nursing is recognized for its many strengths and truly is an integral part of the higher education system.

REFERENCE

Moore, K. M. (1984). The role of mentors in developing leaders for academe. In W. E. Rosenbach & R. L. Taylor (Eds.), *Contemporary issues in leadership* (pp. 209–222). Boulder, CO: Westview Press.

4

The National League for Nursing: Ally or Adversary?

"The League says we have to do it this way." "We can't do that. The League won't allow it." How often have nursing faculty members expressed statements like these? Most of us would have to admit that such comments are not unusual in the academic nursing world.

Statements by nursing faculty members about what "the League" will or will not permit, or what "the League" does or does not require are indicative of several possible situations. They may reflect a lack of understanding about the purposes of the National League for Nursing (NLN) as the organization which accredits nursing programs, the function of accreditation, and just who "the League" is.

Such statements also may indicate a discomfort faculty experience regarding the whole process of being evaluated by their peers. Although faculty members express a value for the evaluation process, stress it as a critical component of the nursing process, and are comfortable (at least to some degree) evaluating student performance, faculty groups often seem to become quite anxious when they and their programs are open to evaluation by the NLN.

Additionally, comments about the power of "the League" also may reflect a faculty group's concern that any feedback from the League that is not positive will jeopardize the status of the nursing program in their institution. Such feedback is viewed as harmful, when it could be most helpful to the program as it attempts to secure additional resources, increase salaries, or heighten the visibility of nursing on campus.

This discussion hopes to clarify the purposes of accreditation, dispel myths about the extent of control the NLN has over nursing curricula and nursing programs, and promote the relationship between the League and various faculty groups as one of allies rather than as one of adversaries. As a result of such understandings, nursing faculty may feel freer to be creative in curriculum approaches and not be as intense and distressed about the accreditation process.

ACCREDITATION PROCESS

Accreditation is a *voluntary* process designed to raise educational standards, strengthen academic curricula, and help faculty maintain a certain level of quality in their programs (*Accreditation and the Future*, 1983; Beckes, 1981; Hawken, 1984). Its origin in higher education in general occurred in the late 1880s with the formation of the New England, Middle States, North Central, and Southwest Associations of Colleges. Medical education initiated steps toward accreditation in the early part of this century and intensified efforts to achieve quality education after the Flexner report (1910).

Nursing's evaluation of the quality of its educational programs had its roots with the Goldmark Report (Committee for the Study of Nursing Education, 1923), and became formalized in 1938 when the National League for Nursing Education initiated a program of accreditation. In 1952, accreditation became a function of the Division of Education of the National League for Nursing, and it has remained within that organization ever since.

Accreditation is a dynamic process through which a nursing program engages in a continuous, systematic evaluation of its educational programs in their totality and in light of the individuality and uniqueness of their parent institution. The specific criteria by which a program is judged are developed by nurse educators involved in similar types of programs (e.g., associate degree or baccalaureate and graduate) and approved by the NLN council which represents those types of programs (e.g., the Councils of Associate Degree or Baccalaureate and Higher Degree Programs). Thus, the standards against which a program is measured are developed and approved by nursing education peers and not by some amorphous, unidentifiable body called "the League" (Chambers, 1983).

The criteria used in evaluating programs (*Criteria for the Evaluation*, 1989, 1990) are intended to serve as standards of quality; as such they are revised periodically to reflect the changing goals and expectations of higher education in general and nursing education in particular. The criteria for the evaluation of baccalaureate and higher degree programs, for example, were revised in 1979, 1983, and again in 1989; shortly after the latest criteria were approved, nurse educators in these programs recognized a need for further refinement to reflect the growing emphasis on the *outcomes* of educational programs, and not merely the *processes* of education. Thus, criteria for evaluation are designed to enhance educational quality and assure program improvement.

In contrast with what many faculty members believe, the criteria for accreditation are quite broad, allowing for creative and unique approaches to designing and implementing curricula. They are far from being narrowly prescriptive, and nursing faculty groups have the freedom to "do their own thing," given there is a sound rationale for the approach and provided it does not violate accepted educational principles (Bear, 1986).

The NLN officers and staff have been responsive to requests from nurse educators for assistance in interpreting the accreditation criteria. Open forums and discussion groups are scheduled at NLN conventions and council meetings, consultants approved by the NLN are available to schools, and manuals to guide the self-study process have been prepared. In this way, faculty groups have the opportunity to seek guidance regarding the criteria and should not feel they have to "go it alone."

Additionally, the NLN membership has recently recommended significant changes in the role of site visitors (giving them greater responsibility to make recommendations about a program's accreditation status), and in the role and composition of the Board of Review (to include a nursing service representative). Such changes were made in response to recommendations from nursing educators and are an attempt to clarify, strengthen, and streamline the accreditation process further.

WHAT IS "THE LEAGUE"?

In one word, the League is *us* — nurse educators as individual members, and nurse educators as representatives of schools of nursing that are members of the NLN (Millard, 1984). In essence, what the League says, the accreditation criteria and procedures it implements (*Policies and Procedures of Accreditation*, 1990), and the standards it sets for educational programs are determined by all members collectively.

One unique feature of the League's membership is that it is open to non-nurses, and, in fact, the Board of Review includes a public member. The input provided by this public member is invaluable because it represents the views of the consumer, thereby bringing a unique dimension to this organization: however, the public members of the NLN and other individual members (even if they are nurse educators) are permitted to vote on all matters *except* accreditation ones. In other words, when accreditation criteria, policies, or procedures are presented for a vote, they are acted on only by the designated representatives of schools of nursing that are themselves accredited.

Site visitors who participate in the accreditation review process are all nurse educators with responsibilities similar to those of faculty at the school being visited, and they usually teach in a type of school similar to the one being evaluated (e.g., a small, liberal arts college). Most Board of Review members also hold academic rank and are actively involved in nursing education programs; the exceptions to this are the one public member and the one nursing service representative. In addition, most NLN professional staff, officers and members of the Board of Governors, are nurse educators, although some may be public members or individual members whose practice is in a service, rather than an academic, setting.

Thus, when the question is asked, "Who is the League?" the best response is, "It's people like you and me." The League is not composed of people from other disciplines or people who are not currently involved in nursing education. Instead, it is composed largely of active nurse educators who are as committed to maintaining the quality and improving the standards of all nursing education programs as are the faculty members teaching in those programs being evaluated.

ACCREDITATION AS AN ENABLING PROCESS

Although many nursing faculty members view the accreditation process as threatening and the relationship between their school of nursing and the NLN as an adversarial one, this need not be so. In fact, when one more clearly understands the purposes of accreditation, the "players" in the accreditation process, and the responsiveness of the NLN to nurse educators' concerns and suggestions about accreditation, the more one can see that the relationship is, in fact, one of alliance.

Almost all programs that undergo a review for NLN accreditation identify areas of weakness as a result of their intensive self-study efforts; and almost all receive some recommendations from the Board of Review regarding how their programs can be enhanced and strengthened to achieve an even greater level of quality. The recognition of such limitations need not be viewed as harmful or "the voice of doom" in terms of the program's future.

Of course, it may be true that some nursing programs may be in financial difficulties or may exist in universities that are not fully supportive of nursing or of professional programs in general. In such institutions, recommendations from the NLN Board of Review addressing the need for more space, increased faculty numbers or salaries, or more current and comprehensive library and laboratory resources to support the nursing program may be received negatively. In fact, the president and board of trustees in this type of institution may respond to such recommendations by suggesting the termination of the nursing program. One might argue, however, that if the nursing program has limited philosophical support and minimal material and human resources in the first place, it may not be able to offer a high-quality educational experience for students, and perhaps it should be terminated. Such is the fate of only a few programs, however.

Most nursing programs, in fact, are able to use the accreditation criteria while they are preparing the self-study report and the recommendations from the Board of Review to their advantage. In an academic institution that values its nursing program and has a commitment to it, the nursing dean or department chair may be able to negotiate successfully for an additional faculty position or more funds to send faculty to professional conferences if the faculty find, during their self-study, that they are not able to provide the individualized instruction they desire or that faculty participation in professional conferences had been limited.

Likewise, in many colleges and universities, the president sees the nursing program as integral to the institution's mission. In such settings, recommendations from the NLN Board of Review that address faculty limitations (e.g., in research and other scholarly activities) may serve to stimulate significant change such as the approval of decreased teaching loads for faculty that provide time for such scholarly efforts. In cases such as these, the nursing dean or department chair may be quite successful in turning the Board of Review recommendations into springboards for new directions and increased resources for the program.

SUMMARY

The process of accreditation—including the critical step of an intensive self-study by a faculty group itself—is an opportunity for faculty to recognize and publicize their strengths, identify their weaknesses or limitations, and set out a plan for building on the former and overcoming the latter (Garner & Chase, 1985). As such, it is and should be a learning experience that promotes growth and quality—an experience that enables faculty to enhance their curricula, clarify relevant policies, affirm their priorities, document their achievements, and identify the directions that future actions need to take.

The NLN and the accreditation process can be strong allies of faculty and administrators in nursing education programs rather than adversaries. As allies, nursing faculty, nursing deans and department chairs, members of the NLN, and all those involved in the accreditation process are working together to continue to strengthen nursing educational programs and improve the standards of quality for nursing programs.

The outcome of such collaboration can be an enhanced power base for nursing faculty groups in their institutions and greater respect for nursing on the university campus. The "winners" of this alliance will be nursing faculty, nursing students, the consumers served by the graduates of our educational programs, employers of our graduates, and the nursing profession itself. It would seem to be an alliance worthy of the effort of each of us.

REFERENCES

Accreditation and the future of quality nursing education. (1983). New York: National League for Nursing.

Bear, E. (1986). Accreditation: Does it control the curriculum? *Journal of Nursing Education, 25*(4), 161–163.

Beckes, I. K. (1981). Toward an understanding of accreditation practices. *Nursing & Health Care, 2*(2), 68–72.

Chambers, C. (1983). *Accreditation and the future of quality of nursing education: What are the standards upon which criteria are based?* New York: National League for Nursing.

Committee for the Study of Nursing Education. (1923). *Nursing and nursing education in the United States.* New York: Macmillan.

Criteria for the evaluation of associate degree programs in nursing (7th ed.). (1990). New York: National League for Nursing.

Criteria for the evaluation of baccalaureate and higher degree programs in nursing (6th ed.). (1989). New York: National League for Nursing.

Flexner, A. (1910). *Medical education in the United States and Canada.* New York: The Carnegie Foundation for the Advancement of Teaching.

Garner, J., & Chase, A. (1985). The accreditation process as a learning experience. *Journal of Nursing Education, 24*(1), 35–37.

Hawken, P. L. (1984). Accreditation: One measure of quality. *Nurse Educator, 9*(1), 20–23.

Millard, R. (1984). The accrediting community: Its members and their interrelations. *Nursing & Health Care, 5*(8), 451–454.

Policies and procedures of accreditation for programs in nursing education (6th ed.). (1990). New York: National League for Nursing.

UNIT II
Thriving in Academe

LETTERS

Dear Terry,

Well, I made the decision to leave the small liberal arts college in which I had been teaching and take a position at the local university. I must admit, the whole job-seeking process and the idea of "selling" myself was easier this time than it was the first time around, but now I find myself presented with an entirely new set of challenges!

Some of those challenges are coming from the expectations the "system" places on more seasoned faculty. And some are coming from me—from my own desires to be promoted in rank, to be awarded tenure, and to do all that is expected of an experienced faculty member.

I must say that when I think about the issue of faculty work load, I do get a bit confused. I was thinking about when I had been job hunting and asked about work load.

One community college chairperson I spoke with was able to show me exactly what constituted a 15-credit-hour semester work load. At one of the private baccalaureate programs where I had interviewed, the chairperson looked quizzically at me when I asked about work load; she said that they really didn't have any specific work-load formula and that I would need to teach a 5-credit-hour course, participate on two nursing department committees and one collegewide committee, advise a complement of 12 to 15 students, and carry out some recruiting activities. When I asked this chairperson about the teacher-student ratio in the classroom, she advised me that there wasn't a limit on enrollment in the nursing courses and there wasn't any money for a teaching assistant, but generally the number of students in any class rarely exceeded 40. When I tried to get specifics on the recruitment activities in which I would be expected to participate, again I received only vague answers.

But there was one aspect of many of the positions I looked into that was very clear: I would get a doctorate, or I would not get tenure!

You know, although my colleagues talk quite a bit about tenure—and promotion—I'm still not sure I really understand the ins and outs of that whole process. Can you shed some light on this for me? I know there are a multitude of responsibilities that must be fulfilled in order to be promoted and obtain tenure. They all appear to be important and necessary hurdles for me at this point in my career, but I *do* wonder how I will ever be able to get it all done and still continue my doctoral studies and spend some time with my family!

I'm hoping you'll be able to help me sort out some of these issues and give some answers. Maybe I'm expecting too much too soon. Please write soon. Your letters always provide me with the insight I know I have but am too reluctant to draw on without some "senior" advice.

Dear Helen,

Once again, your letter resonated with questions and issues that arise daily in academic settings. You seemed a bit surprised to find that work loads, teaching assignments, and faculty expectations are so different from one school to another, but don't be. There are guidelines that the American Association of University Professors (AAUP) publishes about these things, but schools *do* have the freedom to develop systems that work best for them. In fact, the NLN criteria that speak to work load are very broad and allow for flexibility; thus, each school really *does* approach this whole area quite differently.

What you found as *basic* aspects or expectations of a faculty position are quite common: teaching, student advisement, service to the college, service to the community, research, publication, professional involvement, and, in nursing, progress toward or completion of the doctorate. No doubt, it *is* many hats that we wear, and frequently all those roles collide with one another and with our personal lives. It's important to accept, however, that this complexity is part and parcel of a faculty role.

Getting credit and recognition for all these activities also varies from one institution to the next. I've heard of some schools where "points" are given for everything: 2 points for advising 30 students, 4.5 points for teaching a 3-credit course to 51 students (but only 3 points if you teach it to 49 students!), 1.5 points for chairing the curriculum committee (but only 1 point for chairing the faculty development committee), etc. When you reach 12 or 15 points, that's a full-time load. This gets very complicated, but it seems to work well for some schools.

Other schools credit only classroom and clinical teaching, and still others use no formula at all. These latter schools may have some general guidelines (as you said was the case at the baccalaureate school where you had interviewed), but no rigid formula is used. Personally, I like this kind of flexibility, but you need a fair and equitable chairperson to ensure that people don't get abused.

Given the multiple responsibilities a faculty member has, you are going to find *many* times when you'll wonder how in the world you can get it all done. I've been teaching in the university setting for about 18 years, and I still wonder the same thing! Indeed, it seems that as the years go by, I get involved in more projects and committees, and I'm speaking more and providing all kinds of consultation, as well as taking on the mentoring of neophyte nurse educators and writing them long letters. (I must say, though, that this latter role is one I truly enjoy!)

I surely don't have *the* answer to "how to get it all done"—in fact, I don't know if there is *an* answer—but maybe some advice would help. First, I'd say don't underestimate yourself. As a nurse, wife, and mother you have already demonstrated how well you can organize many activities or pieces of information simultaneously. And look how you managed to get through graduate school, work, and raise young children all at the same time. Think about how you managed to accomplish all that, what worked best for you, what your strengths are, and what are the things you don't do very well or don't like to do. Then *use* all these data to devise a game plan.

On the other hand, don't overestimate yourself! Admit that you can't do everything all the time. You have to set priorities and learn how to say "no." (Look at who's telling you to say "no!" I ought to take my own advice!)

Setting priorities, deciding what's important to you and what you value, and knowing when to say "yes" and when to say "no" are easier if you know what your long- and short-term goals are. I know it sounds just like what a teacher would tell a student, but as cliché as it may sound, I have found that looking at goals is a critical step. If one of your children is having difficulty in school and needs your guidance and support now, that becomes a priority; maybe you have to give up running for office in a professional association even though you'd like to be in that position and have a good chance of winning an election. Or if you really want to develop some creative teaching material for your course, then maybe this is not the time to take six doctoral credits; take only three.

On the other hand, if you want to make real progress toward your doctorate, then perhaps you have to decline the chairperson's offer to teach the senior-level issues course (even if it's something you've wanted to do) so you won't have a whole new course to develop. And if promotion and tenure are your goals, then you need to be well aware of the criteria to be met to achieve those goals and concentrate your efforts on meeting those criteria.

All of these decisions are difficult, I know. But then most important decisions *are* difficult. And no matter what choice you make, there are consequences. The thing you need to do is try to anticipate those consequences as best you can and see which ones will best help you meet your personal and professional goals.

Another piece of advice: Remember you are not alone in this world, and you're not the only one with these kinds of problems and concerns. Ask for help if you need it. Seek out your chairperson and faculty colleagues for advice and support. Maybe suggest instituting a doctoral student peer group in your department—an informal forum for all faculty in doctoral programs to gather to support one another, share progress and frustrations, develop "survival tactics," etc. And don't forget me. Call or write any time.

Finally, one last piece of advice I would offer. Get yourself focused. I don't mean to suggest becoming so narrow in your interests that it's limiting. What I *do* mean is, don't be all over the map. If you're teaching an adult health course and want to do some research, why not collaborate with the staff on the clinical units where you take your students to do a small project with their help on a topic that will enhance your teaching as well as address some very real clinical problem? If you want to submit an article for publication, maybe you can do some beginning work on that article through a paper you do in one of your doctoral courses. Or if you are very interested in how students develop as leaders, maybe you can ask to teach in the senior-level leadership course, fulfill a "service to the college" commitment by being the adviser to the student organization, or do some research in that area. The more you can concentrate your efforts, the more efficient you'll be, and you won't feel quite so . . . well . . . schizophrenic!

Well, I have to sign off now because—as you might have guessed—I have 1,001 things to do! But let me give you a word of encouragement. You *can* get it all done and thrive in the process.

I hope I've been of some help. As I said before, why don't we get together soon to go into all of these—and more—issues about career and role development in greater depth. They are critical issues, and it will be helpful to both of us to examine them carefully.

I wish you all the best with your new job and with your efforts in moving toward promotion and tenure. Let me know how it all goes.

5

Faculty Work Load: What It Entails and Getting It All Done

The search is over, the decision is made. The next part of developing a career is to assume the responsibilities inherent in the position accepted. One of the ways to begin this activity is to study the position description and use this as a blueprint for action. Although the emphasis on each area is different from one institution to the next, all faculty positions require a certain amount of teaching, service, and scholarly activity. The position description can provide a guide for how much attention needs to be paid to each of these areas. In addition, information collected from the dean, department chairperson, program director, or level leader will assist in fulfillment of the responsibilities intrinsic to the position.

This chapter will specifically look at the expectations of the role of nurse educator. Unit V will offer insights as to how all of the responsibilities cited in this chapter will ultimately be evaluated by those who administer the program in which one teaches.

TEACHING RESPONSIBILITIES

The primary component of an academic appointment is teaching students. This part of the faculty role consumes approximately 68% of a faculty member's time (Solomons, Jordison, & Powell, 1980). Based on the average faculty member's work week of 54.1 (Solomons, Jordison, & Powell, 1980) to 57.5 hours (Langemo, 1988), the typical nurse educator spends between 36 and 39 hours a week in instruction of students. This figure represents all of the activities that constitute the teaching portion of the faculty role including advising, theory and clinical preparation time, and evaluation, in addition to direct contact hours.

Accepted at some institutions is the formula that states that for every hour of lecture, 2 hours of preparation are necessary (Crawford, Laing, Linwood, Kyle & DeBlock, 1983; Holliman, 1977). If one lectures 3 hours per week, 6 hours of preparation will be needed. In calculating this particular portion of teaching load, a total of 9 hours would be credited toward teaching load, 3 for in-class time, and 6 for preparation.

Some schools of nursing choose to use the team teaching approach to classroom instruction that can confound the application of the preceding described formula. In situations in which team teaching is used in the optimum manner, a group of instructors would present a topic, such as alteration in elimination, from their particular area of expertise. For instance, pediatric, adult health, maternal-child, psychiatric, and gerontological experts would offer content related to alteration in elimination as it presents itself in specific populations. This strategy requires a significant amount of planning but may require less actual presentation time. This strategy is used most in schools that subscribe to an integrated curricula. As one can see, however, use of the formula cited earlier would need some modification.

Clinical time is computed differently by various institutions. College and university policies ordinarily define the laboratory credit for all academic disciplines. In some institutions for every 2 hours of laboratory time, the instructor earns 1 hour of teaching load credit. Others use a 1 to 1, 3 to 1, or a 4 to 1 formula. It is important to determine what the formula is for the institution in which one works.

If, for instance, in College A the nursing faculty position requires 16 hours per week of clinical instruction time, this will count differently depending on the formula used. In a 2 to 1 formula, the faculty member earns 8 teaching hours. In a 3 to 1 formula, the nurse educator earns 5.3 teaching hours. In a 4 to 1 formula, 4 hours are earned. As can be seen, the formula in use by specific colleges and universities can affect the total number of hours earned.

If the program in which one is working uses the 2 to 1 formula to compute clinical load, eight teaching hours are realized for 16 hours of direct clinical supervision, 3 for in-class lecture, and 6 for lecture preparation. The educator earns a total of 17 hours' worth of credit. Crawford, Laing, Linwood, Kyle, and DeBlock (1983) suggest that for every 3 hours of clinical instruction, 1 hour of preparation time should be allocated. Using the data listed earlier, this particular educator earns 5.3 hours of preparation time for 16 hours of clinical instruction. For this example, the total teaching load is 22.3 hours.

The information provided here represents a look at the much debated topic of faculty work load (Courdet, 1981; Crawford et al., 1983; Holliman, 1977; Kirkpatrick, Rose, & Thiele, 1987; O'Shea, 1986; Saylor, Kaylor, Genthe, & Otis, 1979). The teaching aspect of faculty work load is the easiest to compute because the hours spent in these activities are quantifiable. The American Association of University Professors (AAUP) (1970) published a statement on faculty work load. The organization recognized the complexity of developing a statement in light of the myriad "time-consuming institutional duties" (p. 30) required by faculty members but did offer certain guidelines.

Regarding maximum teaching load, the AAUP recommended the following:

> for undergraduate instruction, a teaching load of twelve hours per week, with no more than six separate course-preparations during the academic year. For instruction partly or entirely at the graduate level, a teaching load of nine hours per week. (p. 31)

The pronouncement further stipulated that in offering these guidelines, "it would be misleading to offer this statement without providing some guidelines for a preferable pattern" (p. 31). Preferred work load, according to the AAUP for undergraduate teaching, is 9 hours per week and 6 for graduate.

Using the AAUP guideline, the faculty member in the scenario described earlier would be carrying a teaching overload. Demonstrated here is the necessity of identifying what formula or guidelines the program in which one is employed uses to calculate teaching load. This will help direct the required teaching aspects of the faculty role. It will also provide a measure of what is acceptable and what should not be. Remember, however, that teaching load is only one aspect of work load.

In the situation in which an overload is prescribed for a faculty member for a semester, negotiation can occur to provide for a lighter load in the next semester, or one can negotiate to be paid for the extra load. If a plan to compensate for the overload is not developed, a formal grievance may need to be filed against the institution. As stated in the first chapter, the faculty handbook should provide the new faculty member with information relative to overload compensation, what can and should be grieved, and the mechanism for filing a grievance.

Preparation for Classroom and Clinical Teaching

In preparing for teaching in the classroom or clinical area, the nurse educator should become familiar with a variety of teaching strategies and the media available to support these activities. Initially, allocate time to learn the resources available within the nursing education unit and then explore what resources are available within the college or university. Once the initial time is spent identifying what is available, accessing it will be easier. Preparation is the key to successful teaching.

In addition to preparing for lectures, a faculty member is also responsible for preparing course syllabi and audiovisual materials. These tasks will be easier if one's formal education has included preparation for the teaching role. If not, resources are available in print form to assist in the development of each. Human resources available within the academic unit, such as the curriculum coordinator or someone with a related title, also can be of tremendous help in preparing course-related materials.

In addition, the media specialist within the college or university can provide valuable direction in the preparation of overheads, slides, video recording, and audiotapes. Lectures and seminars can be enhanced by the acquisition and use of these materials.

ADVISEMENT

Another part of the teaching role is the advisement of students. Faculty members surveyed in O'Shea's (1986) study reported that 66% carried 10 or more advisees. Little documentation exists relative to the actual time advisement of an undergraduate student takes. The beginning and end of a semester and registration time are the most labor intensive for faculty. New students, in particular, are likely to consume more faculty time as they make the transition from secondary schooling to college. The new faculty member should establish predetermined office hours to curtail students "dropping in" if unexpected student visits affect one's ability to complete assignments. Although it may be difficult for the new educator to turn a student away, developing an open-door policy during office time limits the ability to begin and complete projects while in the office. One of the greatest challenges to any person in a new position is time management. The nurse educator is no exception.

SERVICE

Provision of service to the academic institution, the community, and the profession is the second major area in which faculty participate. Each one of these areas will be discussed individually to serve as a guide for new faculty members.

Service to the Nursing Department

Rose (1986) directed all faculty to become involved in academic governance. She stated:

> In institutions such as colleges and universities it is not enough to simply perform well in the role of teacher. Faculty members are also expected to participate in the day-to-day work of the organization through the process of academic governance. Educational institutions are governed jointly by administration and faculty, with faculty taking a very real part in organizational decision-making. (p. 8)

Thus, it behooves the new faculty member to learn as much as possible about the governance of a particular institution and how one can become involved in it.

In the nursing department, several types of committees exist universally: curriculum, student affairs, and faculty affairs. Any number of other committees may exist given the particular needs of the department. For instance, many programs have recruitment committees to develop strategies for enhancing the number of qualified applicants to the program. In some instances, the governance of the department or college of nursing requires that groups such as a recruitment group be developed as a task force rather than as a standing committee. Reference to the nursing department's policies and procedures or bylaws will direct new faculty members about this and related activities.

In 1987 de Tornyay delineated the types of committees found in nursing departments into three categories: policy making, administrative, and technical. Policy-making committees "develop regulations and criteria for academic activities" (p. 5). Administrative committees use the guidelines developed by the policy-making committees to make administrative decisions related to the program's function. An example of an administrative committee using de Tornyay's perspective is the admissions committee. Finally, the last type described by de Tornyay is the technical committee. This committee "provides technical advice to faculty and administration" (p. 5). A function of this type of committee might be the evaluation of personal computer equipment. All of the committees described offer valuable service to the nursing department. For the department to run efficiently and effectively it is necessary for faculty to contribute their time and effort to this part of their role.

Service to the Institution

In addition to functioning on committees and task forces within the nursing department, there is also the expectation that faculty members participate in college and university governance. This is on a larger scale than the department and places the faculty member in an excellent position to contribute to the present and future direction taken by the institution. Similar to the nursing department, many of the committees at the college or university level deal with issues related to student and faculty affairs. Policy-making and policy-enforcing committees exist to ensure the smooth operation of the organization. The following is noted by Kritek (1985):

> Faculty governance is predicated on the assumption that the mission of the university, the generation and transmission of knowledge, is the responsibility of faculty, the professional community of scholars. Faculty governance assures professional autonomy, the freedom to control central educational tasks and professional activities. (p. 357)

In carrying out this activity, new faculty members interested in participating on a particular college or university committee should inform their dean or department chair of their interest and ask that their names be submitted for membership. It may also be useful to introduce oneself to the committee chairperson and verbalize interest in membership. Generally, new faculty members limit their participation in governance to departmental committees during their first year; they usually would become involved in academic governance at the broader level later in their careers. During the first year, one has the opportunity to "settle into" the new role and the demands it places on personal time and resources before becoming involved beyond the nursing department.

When the time comes to become a member of a college or university committee, it is useful, if possible, to select committees that are congruent with one's personal interests or which have goals and objectives similar to committees on which one participates in the nursing department. Choosing committees with similar goals and objectives will narrow the scope of activities necessary to be an effective member of each group.

Professional Service

Added to responsibilities of academic governance is the necessity of participating in professional organizations. Many individuals will develop professional affiliations before becoming nurse educators. Individuals who become members of the American Nurses' Association or other nursing practice groups on entry into the nursing profession often move toward assuming roles in governance of those organizations during their tenure with the organization.

Functioning effectively as a nurse educator demands a tremendous time commitment to fulfill all the expectations of the role. Thus, it is necessary to choose professional organizational involvement carefully. Early in one's career a nurse educator may choose to be a committee member, move on to a chair position, and later run for an elected office. As suggested earlier, pooling one's interest will facilitate effective use of time.

In addition to developing in the role of nurse educator, individuals also should be focusing on the career goals that were developed before assuming the first position. Participating in professional organizations is an excellent way to advance one's career, but as stated earlier, one would be wise to choose commitments and level of involvement carefully.

Community Service

Provision of service to the community in which one lives may also be an expectation in institutions whose mission includes such activities. If this is the case, it will be important to select a community group in which one's activities will support movement toward career goals. As a rule, institutions of higher education do not define the community groups with which one should serve. Considered in one's choice should be how to make the most out of a commitment while fulfilling the requirements for promotion and tenure. For instance, on many campuses Special Olympics Programs are coordinated by faculty and students and held on college and university athletic fields. By volunteering to be available to provide first aid, the nurse educator is providing a community service by using his or her nursing expertise. Functioning in this capacity will require the time commitment only on the days of the event. As repeatedly suggested here, finding ways to pool resources will enable the educator to meet the demands of the role with the least amount of difficulty.

SCHOLARSHIP

One of the responsibilities of a learned profession is to advance the body of knowledge respective to the particular discipline. Nurses educated beyond the basic educational preparation have a responsibility to be a part of knowledge generation, use, and dissemination in the field. This professional expectation can be met in the development of a research agenda, an area of concern particularly for faculty teaching in senior colleges and universities.

Development of a Research Agenda

Initially, the neophyte nurse educator may be part of a research team or develop pilot projects in an area of interest. Using a research mentor either on the faculty where one is teaching or external to the organization is an excellent way to begin a research career. New faculty should negotiate for resources to begin exploration of topics of interest that are important to the discipline before being hired. Holzemer and Chambers's (1988) research on faculty productivity revealed that faculty members who spend more time on research have more publications, higher academic rank, and greater numbers of funded research projects; thus, they were viewed as being more productive faculty members. They also state the following:

> Newly prepared research faculty may wish to think carefully about accepting a position where they would become "the" researchers, as opposed to joining a group of well-established faculty where they would be assuming a "junior" faculty role and where their own productivity may be nurtured. (p. 17)

University settings will continue to expect nurse faculty involvement in research; however, in liberal arts colleges and junior colleges, the expectation for research may be less. In these institutions the emphasis is generally on the quality of instruction rather than on research. Depending on one's personal career agenda, one type of academic setting may be chosen over the other as the first employment setting.

As one's career advances and the goal of promotion or tenure is viewed as a short-term goal, it will be necessary to develop a clearly defined research agenda. A plainly stated direction for research along with an outline of studies one wishes to carry out related to a field of interest will provide direction. Once an agenda has been designed, the nurse educator will be required to take a leadership role in research project development.

Grant Writing

In line with research activities will be the expectation that grants be written to support the defined research objectives. Similar to the role one plays in developing research, it is considered appropriate initially to be part of a grant-writing team and, as time goes on, to move into the principal investigator role in areas of interest.

In addition to writing grants to support one's own research agenda, one also may be expected to write grants that will support program expansion. An example of a grant to support program expansion would be one that focuses on the addition of a new concentration within an existing master's program. This type of grant writing is particularly expected when the nurse educator's master's or doctor's education has been in the area of curriculum development or nursing education. When opportunities present themselves to be part of any type of grant-writing experience, the new nurse educator would be wise to agree to be involved, even if only peripherally.

Publication

In addition to conducting research and writing grants, scholarly production is required in the area of publication. The old "publish or perish" challenge has a great deal of truth to it, depending on the institution in which one is employed. Tenure and promotion committees frequently look at the types of publications, such as opinion, how-to, or research articles, where they have been published, and what the applicant's authorship role is in the publication.

Once completed, there is an expectation that the findings of one's research study will be published. Writing about what one has done is difficult for some and less so for others. Various reference materials, however, are available to assist in the development of research articles. One of the better ways to begin writing is the use of a "publishing" mentor. Often the first prepared manuscript is rejected. With the help of a mentor, one can critically and objectively examine the work with another who is not invested in the work. The mentor can provide the novice writer with suggestions for a revision, encouragement throughout the rewriting phase, and support when the acceptance or rejection letter arrives. Williams and Blackburn (1988) found in their research that the mentor can protect the mentee from nonproductive time-consuming activities.

In addition to publishing research, there is often the opportunity to write about innovative teaching strategies, new clinical developments, faculty projects, or personal nursing experiences. Many of the ideas held by new educators are ones not written about yet. One of the advantages of being a new instructor is the discovery of information about topics that are unfamiliar. While doing this investigation, the neophyte will discover the "holes" in the literature. The "holes" in the literature can be filled by those who discover them. This challenge is available to the new nurse educator.

Other publishing opportunities that can be pursued include authoring a column for a local newspaper, a chapter for a book, or a book on nursing or a health-related subject. Although these activities are generally not refereed, meaning that they do not undergo a blind review by scholars in your field as to their importance, and therefore may not be recognized as having a high degree of scholarship, they do reflect one's interest in and commitment to publishing.

Presentations

Finally, in relation to scholarship, faculty members are responsible for presenting their research ideas. As stated earlier, a learned profession is obligated to continue developing the body of knowledge specific to the discipline. Research alone is not enough. Nurse academicians are expected to share the knowledge they hold with others in the profession. In addition to publishing the newly discovered information, nurse scholars can share their knowledge through presentation of it.

A myriad of possible ways to present information exists. Similar to publication, some kinds of presentation are viewed as more prestigious and will hold more "power" in promotion and tenure decisions. For instance, presenting at a national or international conference will be viewed as more prestigious than a presentation for a local nurse practice group. As a new teacher it may be necessary to start on a smaller scale and develop expertise in presentations before moving on to regional, national, or international conferences.

Nurse educators have a clear advantage over other nurses in the area of presenting. By virtue of the activities involved in transmitting knowledge to students, educators have the public speaking experience unknown to most nurses.

Presentations can initially be offered to groups of colleagues. The new nurse educator may be asked or volunteer to share an innovative teaching strategy. Sharing this information with a group of faculty may start a list of speaking engagements. Offering to explain a new clinical development at a professional meeting is another way to begin a speaking career.

Ultimately, the goal is to present research, theoretical developments, or clinical information to state, national, or international audiences. Submissions of abstracts for large assemblies is generally required.

Presentation of knowledge is an expectation for those holding academic appointments in institutions of higher learning. Development as a nurse educator scholar will move one's career as well as meeting the expectations of the role. Presenting speeches, symposia, and seminars by abstract submission will eventually lead to invited presentations that are considered the sine qua non of public speaking in the academic world.

SUMMARY

In this chapter the various aspects of the nurse educator role have been examined. The nurse educator must be a teacher, adviser, researcher, author, and public speaker as well as serve the college or university, profession, and community. All of this is possible if one takes the time to plan and choose carefully the activities in which one becomes involved and the routes to meeting these requirements. Pooling resources and using a mentor are two good ways of developing a strong base as a developing academician. Teaching is an excellent way to affect the future of the profession. Many individuals choose teaching as a career every year. Careful planning and gradual building of expertise in all parts of the role will provide the neophyte educator with the desired career outcomes.

REFERENCES

American Association of University Professors (1970). Statement on faculty workload. *AAUP Bulletin, 56,* 30–32.

Courdet, N. A. (1981). Determining faculty workload. *Nurse Educator, 6*(2), 38–41.

Crawford, M. E., Laing, G., Linwood, M., Kyle, M., & DeBlock, A. (1983). A formula for calculating faculty workload. *Journal of Nursing Education, 22*(7), 285–286.

de Tornyay, R. (1987). Too many committees? *Journal of Nursing Education, 26*(1), 5.

Holliman, J. M. (1977). Analyzing faculty workload. *Nursing Outlook, 25*(11), 721–723.

Holzemer, W. L., & Chambers, D. B. (1988). A contextual analysis of faculty productivity. *Journal of Nursing Education, 27*(1), 10–18.

Kirkpatrick, M. K., Rose, M. A., & Thiele, R. (1987). Faculty workload measures: The time is right. *Journal of Nursing Education, 26*(2), 84–86.

Kritek, P. B. (1985). Faculty governance: A key to professional autonomy. *Journal of Nursing Education, 24*(9), 356–359.

Langemo, D. V. (1988). Work-related stress in baccalaureate nurse educators. *Western Journal of Nursing Research, 10*(3), 327–334.

O'Shea, H. S. (1986). Faculty workload: Myths and realities. *Journal of Nursing Education, 25*(1), 20–25.

Rose, M. A. (1986). Managing your academic career. Academic governance: You must get involved. *Nurse Educator, 13*(3), 8–9.

Saylor, A. A., Kaylor, L. E., Genthe, D., & Otis, E. (1979). *American Journal of Nursing, 79*(5), 902–904.

Solomons, H. C., Jordison, N. S., & Powell, S. R. (1980). How faculty members spend their time. *Nursing Outlook, 28*(3), 160–165.

Williams, R., & Blackburn, R. T. (1988). Mentoring and junior faculty productivity. *Journal of Nursing Education, 27*(5), 204–209.

6

Promotion and Tenure

Promotion and tenure. The mere words often cause faculty members, especially relatively new faculty members, to pale and to question their competence. "Can I *ever* do all that I need to do to be promoted or to get tenure?" is a question often asked by faculty members. In addition, many wonder if their career in academe will be abruptly terminated when the time to apply for promotion and tenure arrives.

Faculty, therefore, often view promotion and tenure as obstacles in their career paths. These phenomena, which are unique to the world of higher education, can be seen as opportunities to challenge oneself to grow professionally and to make significant contributions to one's field, however. Perhaps the fear that so many faculty members have about promotion and tenure comes from a lack of understanding about these processes; this discussion serves to enhance nursing faculty's knowledge in this area.

ACADEMIC RANKS

In the university setting, faculty may be appointed to one of several ranks. Typically, those ranks, in ascending order of progression, are instructor, assistant professor, associate professor, and professor. Each rank expects a higher level of accomplishment than the previous one, and the upper ranks (i.e., associate professor and professor) may be reserved for individuals who, in addition to having met the teaching and scholarship criteria, have served in the preceding rank for a specified number of years.

Instructor

The instructor rank generally is given to individuals with no or minimal teaching experience in an academic setting and who hold the master's degree in nursing. Some universities and some disciplines that require the doctorate for appointment to a university faculty position may award the rank of instructor to a doctorally prepared individual with little or no previous experience; however, in nursing, this rank typically is awarded to individuals without doctoral degrees. In many instances, instructors are expected to concentrate their efforts on developing their teaching expertise and increasing their "service" involvement at the department level and in the profession.

Assistant Professor

For those nursing faculty members who hold the doctorate and have little or no teaching experience at the university level, or who hold the master's degree but have had several years of teaching in senior colleges, the rank of assistant professor may be awarded. Assistant professors frequently are expected to be capable teachers and individuals who have been involved in their professional organizations and their departments. In their new rank, they are expected to maintain these contributions while increasing their service involvement at the university level and developing their research and scholarship skills.

Associate Professor

After successfully holding the rank of assistant professor for several years (typically three to six years), an individual may be promoted to the rank of associate professor. Associate professors generally are seasoned teachers who have demonstrated excellence in that area, individuals who have contributed in sustained ways to their profession and to the academic institutions in which they have been involved, and scholars who have contributed to their field in significant ways. At the associate professor rank, individuals are expected to be actively involved in all the dimensions of a faculty role—teaching, service, and scholarship—and provide leadership within their university and their academic discipline.

Professor

The highest rank to which faculty members can be appointed or promoted is that of professor, sometimes referred to as full professor to distinguish it from the other two professorial ranks. Individuals are generally promoted to the rank of professor after having successfully held the rank of associate professor for 5 to 10 years, depending on the institution's policies, and after having achieved distinction in their field through research and other scholarly activities. Those who hold this rank also have demonstrated excellence in teaching and have been consistent in service contributions.

WHAT DOES PROMOTION INVOLVE?

The specific process for promotion in rank is determined by each institution and, thus, varies from one university to the next. The process, however, generally is characterized by five aspects: (a) The process is initiated by individuals when they believe they have met the criteria for the next rank; (b) applications for promotion can be made only for the next rank (e.g., instructor to assistant professor, not instructor to associate professor); (c) a packet of material supporting the application for promotion accompanies the request; (d) the application material is reviewed by the individual's faculty peers and dean or department chairperson, who make recommendations; and (e) for promotion to the upper two ranks, the application packet is subject to review by an interdisciplinary, university-wide committee or external reviewers.

Faculty members considering applying for promotion in rank would do well to discuss the specifics of the institution's policies, criteria, and procedures with the dean or department chairperson. In some schools, the department's promotion and tenure committee members also may be available for guidance and consultation. Seeking such guidance is quite helpful to candidates who wish to submit strong, relevant, well-documented applications for promotion.

The application packet itself may vary in its specific contents, but it typically includes evidence regarding the individual's accomplishments. The new faculty member should begin early to create a filing system for materials that may eventually be included in a promotion application packet.

Materials to include in a promotion application packet may include but not be limited to the following: student evaluations of teaching, peer evaluations of teaching, programs of professional meetings at which papers were presented, lists of all courses taught including dates and number of students in class for each, letters of appreciation and recognition from students or colleagues or conference organizers, and lists of all committees on which one has served including dates and particular contributions made to the committee's work. In addition, one may be expected to include copies of all publications, letters of acceptance of manuscripts if one's publication has not yet appeared in print, letters of acceptance of a paper for presentation if the conference has not yet occurred, lists of all professional conferences and meetings attended, the number and type of students advised, and any special projects completed or contributed to for the department or university.

Keeping all promotion material on file and organized serves several purposes: (a) It reinforces all that has been accomplished and helps individuals evaluate when they are "ready" to seek promotion; (b) it is more easily compiled when the time comes to submit the application packet; and (c) it provides more objective evidence of a variety of ways in which the promotion criteria have been met. Thus, a strong, well-supported application, which is well organized, is put forth for review.

Faculty members who are being considered for promotion in rank generally prepare a packet that documents their accomplishments since their appointment to their current rank, even if some of those occurred while at another institution. In contrast, individuals being considered for tenure usually are judged on their achievements while at the college or university where they are seeking tenure.

Usually the packet that the candidate has compiled for promotion is reviewed by the departmental promotion and tenure committee, which makes a recommendation on the application. This recommendation may be made to the department chair, dean, university-wide committee, academic vice-president, or other individual or body, depending on the institution's policy. The candidate's department chair or dean also makes a recommendation, which may be included with or separate from that of the committee, and which also is forwarded to the appropriate individual or group.

In many institutions, the department promotion and tenure committee and the dean or department chair's recommendations regarding promotion from instructor to assistant professor are sent to the academic vice-president, who acts on it. Such applications may not be reviewed by the interdepartmental promotion and tenure committee, particularly in large universities.

Applications for promotion to the upper ranks, however, usually undergo an internal review at the department level and by a university-wide committee, the latter of which is frequently composed of tenured associate professors and professors from a variety of disciplines. These applications also may undergo external reviews.

External reviewers usually are tenured faculty who hold the rank at or above that to which the candidate is applying and who teach at schools comparable with the candidate's. They are asked (a) whether this candidate would be granted promotion in their institution, given the content of the application packet, and (b) to comment on the quality of the applicant's contributions to her or his field, particularly in the area of research.

The comments of the external reviewers, if such reviewers are used, along with the entire application packet and the recommendations of the departmental committee and the candidate's chair or dean are reviewed by the university-wide promotion and tenure committee. Ultimately, all recommendations are forwarded for final action to the academic vice-president, university president, or board of trustees, depending on the institution's policies. Candidates are then notified of the decision regarding their application.

WHAT IS TENURE?

Tenure is a system that was advocated by the American Association of University Professors (AAUP) in the early part of this century, primarily as a means to protect faculty members' academic freedom, that is, their right to teach various ideas and points of view freely and without censure. In essence, tenure is an unwritten "contract" between a faculty member and a university in which the individual makes a commitment to the university to remain as a contributing member of the faculty, and the institution assures the faculty member a position for life, provided no extraordinary circumstances arise.

According to the AAUP ("Academic Freedom and Tenure," 1963), tenure is a means to two primary ends: (a) freedom of teaching, research, and extramural activities; and (b) a sufficient degree of economic security to make teaching attractive. It typically is granted after a probationary period of no more than 7 years and after a rigorous peer review.

The process of applying for tenure is similar to that of applying for promotion to the upper ranks: the individual initiates the process, an application packet containing the same material is prepared, the application is reviewed internally by the departmental promotion and tenure committee as well as by the candidate's chair or dean and the university-wide promotion and tenure committee, and, depending on the university's policy, the application may be sent to external reviewers. The one significant difference between the processes of applying for promotion and applying for tenure is that candidates cannot wait to submit an application for tenure until they believe they are "ready"; they must submit it within the designated period.

In most instances, although individuals may apply for tenure in less than the typical 7-year probationary period, they may not extend that period. Individuals who are in or moving into their sixth or seventh year of a tenure-track position must apply for tenure or accept the fact that if an application is not made or is not reviewed positively, their position will no longer be available after the seventh year.

In some universities, the criteria and procedures for tenure and promotion to the rank of associate professor are so closely related that the two are almost synonymous. In other words, when individuals apply for promotion to the rank of associate professor, they also must apply for tenure. The criteria for both must be met simultaneously, and both are awarded concurrently. Thus, faculty members need to be fully aware of the promotion and tenure policies in their institution to ensure that their reviews will be most successful (Freeman & Voigner, 1985).

NONTENURE TRACK LINES

Tenure has been criticized sharply by many in higher education (Walden, 1980) for "guaranteeing" jobs for life in a way no other type of institution does, protecting the incompetent, being based on a subjective and informal review process, retaining "deadwood" faculty, and "protect[ing] everything but death, retirement, or assassinating a member of the Board of Trustees" (Moog, 1972, p. 131). In light of such criticisms, a number of institutions have chosen to abolish the tenure system, and others have followed different options.

Some universities have moved to offering multiple (5 to 10) year contracts to employees who have consistently served the university well and whom they wish to keep as viable members of their faculty (Bueche, 1983; Fleming, 1983). Other institutions have implemented approaches to decrease the subjectivity that seems to be inherent in tenure reviews (Saaty & Ramanujam, 1983). Still other universities have other options for faculty appointments, such as nontenure track appointments or clinical track appointments, neither of which would end in tenure or the "lifelong" commitment between the faculty member and the institution.

Nursing faculty who are engaged in doctoral study, wish to pursue a stronger clinical focus, or are unable to commit to all the professional and scholarly requirements of a regular faculty role at a particular point in their lives may choose to opt for or negotiate a nontenure track position. This would provide the time needed to work toward meeting the criteria for promotion and tenure.

CONSIDERATIONS FOR THE INDIVIDUAL NURSING FACULTY MEMBER

It is, perhaps, obvious from the preceding discussion that meeting the criteria for promotion in rank or for tenure is a challenging process that puts great demands on the individual. It can be a frightening, overwhelming process, particularly to the novice nurse educator, the faculty member who takes a position with minimal or no preparation or background in teaching, or the teacher who joins a university faculty without holding the doctorate.

Fewer than 20 years ago, many in nursing education argued that the master's degree was the terminal degree and that faculty should be appointed as assistant professors, promoted to the upper ranks, or tenured even if they did not hold the doctorate, or if they had made minimal or no scholarly contributions. This argument was based on the facts that there were few master's-prepared nurses available, doctoral study in nursing was extremely limited, and the development of the body of nursing knowledge had barely begun.

Since that time, however, the number of master's-prepared nurses, although still limited, has grown tremendously, doctoral study in nursing and for nurses has become more available and accessible, there has been great progress in developing nursing science and in nurses' scholarly efforts, and the profession has set higher standards for itself. As a result, nurse educators now wish to hold parity with their faculty colleagues in other disciplines. Nurse educators have explicated the doctorate as the terminal degree in nursing, just as is the case in other fields, and they expect to be held to the same criteria for promotion and tenure as all other faculty (Murphy, 1985).

Nurse educators who assume faculty positions without the doctorate may be wise to negotiate for nontenure track positions, as previously described, if they are available options. If such options are not possible, however, faculty may choose to use their time on a tenure track line as an opportunity to develop their teaching expertise and gain experience working on various department and collegewide committees while they complete the doctorate.

In today's academic environment, it is unreasonable to expect to receive tenure in one's first teaching position. Thus, novice educators may wish to embark on their teaching careers in schools that present fewer pressures for scholarly activities, emphasize teaching, are slower paced, allow one to complete doctoral studies, and give the time and experience needed to secure another position in the future. In fact, one may even be promoted to the rank of assistant professor during this initial appointment and, therefore, be in a better position when pursuing one's next appointment.

As mentioned in the discussion of securing a faculty appointment, faculty members' long- and short-term goals are important guides throughout their careers, and this is true particularly in relation to promotion and tenure. Individuals whose ultimate goal is to teach in a research university will need to use promotion and tenure expectations to guide their efforts. They may focus their efforts on developing teaching skills under the guidance of a colleague who successfully combines teaching and research, fulfilling their service commitments by serving on university and professional committees that focus on research, and entering into mentor relationships with those in the field with similar scholarly interests In this way, promotion and tenure can be viewed as opportunities to facilitate professional growth and meet long-range goals, not merely as obstacles or roadblocks.

Conversely, individuals may wish to focus their careers on developing excellence in teaching. Such persons may choose to accept faculty appointments in liberal arts colleges, junior colleges, or universities dedicated to teaching, focus their research efforts on teaching and learning, and invest their professional efforts in projects and committees that address educational issues and concerns.

SUMMARY

Promotion and tenure, although challenging processes, need not be the overwhelming, devastating experiences many faculty members believe them to be. Instead, they can be seen as opportunities to challenge individuals to strive toward higher standards, concentrate their efforts so that long-term goals can be achieved, and seek review of their accomplishments by peers.

It is important to remember, however, that once appointment to the upper ranks and tenure are achieved, one has the responsibility to continue to grow and be an excellent teacher, scholar, and contributor to one's discipline and university. Such an honor is not a license to "sit back and do nothing," or an invitation to "rest on one's laurels." Rather, it is a challenge to excel and to serve as a mentor and guide to neophyte nurse educators.

REFERENCES

Academic freedom and tenure: 1940 statement of principles. (1963). *AAUP Bulletin, 49,* 192–193.

Bueche, M. M. (1983). Academic tenure: A re-examination for the eighties. *Nurse Educator, 8*(1), 3–8.

Fleming, J. W. (1983). Tenure today. *American Journal of Nursing, 83*(2), 279–280.

Freeman, L. H., & Voigner, R. R. (1985). Clarifying tenure requirements. *Nursing Outlook, 33*(1), 43–45.

Moog, F. (1972). Tenure is obsolete. In D. W. Vermilye (Ed.), *The expanded campus* (pp. 130–136). San Francisco: Jossey-Bass.

Murphy, M. I. (1985). A descriptive study of faculty tenure in baccalaureate and graduate programs in nursing. *Journal of Professional Nursing, 1*(1), 14–22.

Saaty, T. L., & Ramanujam, V. (1983). An objective approach to faculty promotion and tenure by the analytic hierarchy process. *Research in Higher Education, 18*(3), 311–331.

Walden, T. (1980). Tenure: A review of the issue. *Educational Forum, 44*, 363–372.

UNIT III
Providing Quality Education

LETTERS

DEAR TERRY,

I find it hard to believe that the time has come for me to assume the responsibility for developing and contracting student learning experiences. During my first year, I was getting myself together, trying to learn as much as I could about this place and hoping that some wisdom would descend from the heavens and make me a better teacher. Now that I've had the time and opportunity to get into the thick of things I find it necessary to re-assess some ideologies and "sacred cows" held by nurse educators in general (maybe all nurses) and some specific ones here.

The primary teaching methodology used by me and most of the other faculty here is what is called lecture-discussion. When examined closely however, I find that it is more lecture-comment. There appears to be a per-vasive feeling that you cannot cover all of the material that the students need for "boards" without lecturing. I must admit that at some intellectual level I accept this. I know that I shouldn't, but there is a price for creativity, and I'm not sure that the cost is always worth the time investment. Wow! I can't believe I just wrote that! I was so full of idealism when I left graduate school, and now I have the feeling that I've sold out to mediocrity. There must be some way to help me with this attitude. Possibly, if I can offer a weak excuse it might have something to do with the overwhelming responsibilities I have here. I think I need to digress a little to illustrate my thoughts.

As I'm very sure you are aware, there is the responsibility for evaluation of students. Evaluation measures must be prepared, administered, and scored, which takes a tremendous amount of time. Then, of course, there are frequent meetings with those students whose progress is slow or nonexistent. I feel a tremendous duty to evaluate every piece of student-generated data at least twice to make sure that I am being the absolute fairest I can be. Aside from that, there is the requirement to evaluate and reevaluate evaluation measures that I have developed. In addition, I try to obtain evaluation measures used by other faculty to see that mine are similar in structure and not needlessly repetitive in their focus.

Another responsibility I have is to remain credible among my other colleagues within the institution. I participate on several committees that are very active. In some instances, the committee meets weekly or bimonthly with individual assignments to be completed in the interim. In addition there is the imperative to present workshops, papers, and do research. I also have the requisite of completing the doctorate, a burden many of my colleagues in other departments were smart enough to complete prior to their entrance into academia.

Negotiating student learning experiences within the clinical setting is another one of the important functions of the position. Inherent in this is the obscure responsibility for maintaining relations with the affiliating clinical institution. I must admit that I believed that all of the service-education rhetoric was an attempt on the part of graduate faculties to keep their respective programs competing. I no longer believe it. Now that I live in the "real world," I find that the missions of the service setting and the educational setting *are* in some instances at opposite ends of the spectrum. I frequently find myself discussing at length with other faculty the absurdity of taking students in at 7 A.M. just so that the nurses' routines are not upset. I am, however, all too aware of how hostile the environment can become on a clinical unit if the nurses are asked to alter their routines too much to conform to students' learning experiences and schedules. I must admit that most of the time I'm willing to forgo the argument in the negotiation of clinical experiences so that I am able to optimize the students' learning experience by having staff nurses available who do not resent their (the students') presence (intrusion?).

Another little problem related to this same issue is how to teach the implementation of nursing theory in an environment that supports another model, or one that subscribes to a model at the administrative level but functions without one at the unit level. I don't want to sound like I'm dumping on the staff nurses because I'm not. I know that most of them are lucky if they have time to go to the bathroom during the day. I feel very distressed over what is happening in hospitals—too many business managers and not enough individuals to interpret the realities. You and I have had this discussion many times, but I don't believe that clients are part of "product lines," a management concept that affects all aspects and all levels of nursing practice these days.

I guess I've digressed enough from my original discussion, that being, why I don't have time for creative teaching strategies. After writing all of my excuses why I haven't found time to be creative I find myself even more convinced that the time I do have available to develop creative strategies is at a premium. But I *do* think it is important for me to find that time to be creative and to ensure that students get a quality education. I hope you can help me put my responsibilities in perspective so that I can use my talents in the best possible way. Write soon and give my regards to our mutual associates.

DEAR HELEN,

Your most recent letter truly "hit home" because I had just been engaged in a rather intense discussion with one of my colleagues about the whole issue of providing quality education. You see, it seems to me that in too many instances nurse educators have settled for mediocrity and given up on striving for excellence. I know that sounds like I'm saying the whole world is "going to pot," and I don't mean to imply that. I really do believe, however, that the general attitude—no matter where you go—is "Let's do what we have to do to get by and not one thing more." It seems to me, however, that in the professional areas of *our* lives—teaching and nursing care—that's not good enough!

Sure, there are days when you just don't feel like "giving it your all" and times when you just can't be overly creative and excited about the class you're teaching. Nursing faculty members are human beings just like anyone else! When those kinds of days come to be the norm instead of the exception, though, then I begin to worry.

My experience in teaching has been just like what you describe. The most common teaching strategy used is lecture-comment, the overwhelming concern about "teaching what students need to know to pass boards" is evident, and the willingness of many faculty to invest the time and energy to make teaching and learning fun and exciting is minimal. I think you are right in making a connection between those circumstances and the overwhelming responsibilities nursing faculty members have. It also seems to me that at some point, those circumstances evolve into excuses. The outcome of all this is that faculty members stagnate, students "plod" through programs but are not excited about nursing or what they are learning, and the products of our education programs are not the professional change agents desired. The final result is that nursing suffers.

When I think of the issue of providing quality education, so many things come to my mind. I think of our elaborate, carefully constructed curriculum designs and the painfully constructed conceptual frameworks and level objectives. I think about the literally hundreds of teaching strategies we can use to help students learn, to make teaching more fun, and to enhance creativity, and I reflect on the fact that many of these strategies have been shown through research to be more effective than traditional strategies. I think about the sophisticated mechanisms we have developed to evaluate students (and all aspects of programs) to ensure that objectives are being met. I think of the expertise of the faculty, their abilities as clinicians, and their abilities as teacher. I think of the relationships we have with so many diverse clinical facilities that provide valuable learning experiences for students. Also, I think about the relationships that develop between nursing students and nursing faculty that rarely evolve in other disciplines.

There's no doubt that the issue of providing quality education in nursing is a complex one. Most faculty members express a desire to provide quality education, but what happens in reality? For whatever reasons, faculty members often seem to ignore the framework and don't use it to guide their teaching and selection of learning experiences. Faculty members seem to think level objectives have no relation to the courses that are being taught. There are arguments that creative teaching strategies take excessive time to develop and an unreasonable amount of class time to use. Faculty members seem unable or unwilling to identify themselves as faculty instead of clinicians and attempt to be both, with the result being that they try to maintain excellence in two different spheres of practice and often end up not being expert in either one. There seems to be a divisive force that exists between education and service instead of a cooperative and collaborative one. Finally, we seem to forget that we have such unique relationships with our students. It seems to me that if we addressed some of these areas, the quality of what we do would be enhanced tremendously.

You're well aware, I know, of the numerous studies that have been done recently about the quality of higher education in general. The criticisms that have been leveled against higher education are that students cannot read or write at a level once expected of a college graduate, have no awareness of their history or the world around them, and cannot think. Criticisms also abound that professional schools prepare people for jobs but do not prepare educated men and women. These comments are not, of course, limited to nursing programs, and nursing faculty can feel good about that. At the same time, however, nursing programs are not immune to such critiques, and that cannot be ignored.

I understand fully when you say there is a price for creativity and the cost sometimes is not worth the results, and I know the tremendous work load nursing faculty carry. On the other hand, I also am convinced that if we continue to meet *our* needs instead of those of our *students*, the day may come when we no longer have students to teach.

Possibly faculty don't implement the conceptual framework effectively because they don't know what the framework really is or what it is supposed to do. Perhaps they don't know enough about a variety of teaching strategies, and the thought of using something that is not as "controlled" as lecture is frightening and overwhelming. Maybe they are afraid that if they don't cover every piece of information on a subject in class students will not pass boards, and someone will come back pointing a finger at *them* saying they didn't do their job well enough. It might even be the case that nurse educators are unable to negotiate more valuable clinical learning experiences because the resources available to the staff nurses in the agencies are too depleted and cannot be compensated for by a faculty member.

I wonder if part of the problem is that because there *are* so many aspects to the issues of quality education, faculty members think they cannot possibly solve all the problems so they end up not trying to solve any of them. If you want to develop creative teaching strategies for a course, don't try to do something exceptional for every class all in one semester. Take *one* class session, develop it in a creative way, evaluate its success, and revise it as needed for the next time around; in the next semester, take another class session and develop *it* in a creative way. No one expects you to do it all at once.

Possibly your faculty needs to institute some open forums to discuss just what is meant by quality education and then take a long, hard, careful look at the extent to which it is being provided. My guess is that by listening to what students say about their classes and clinical experiences and the suggestions they make for improvements, you will find that many of them can be accommodated quite reasonably. They might even make teaching more fun for you! Students *do* respond positively to different formats for class, and they *do* have some very good ideas about what would be beneficial for them in the clinical area. They may not be sophisticated in curriculum design and teaching-learning principles, but they *do* know what works for them and what excites them. We should listen and respond to that more.

Remember when we talked about faculty work load? I suggested you try not to take on all the aspects of the faculty role at the same time. It seems to me the same advice is appropriate when it comes to providing quality education.

If each faculty member could begin to develop strategies to enhance the educational experience from one aspect of interest, eventually the whole problem would be tackled. When one faculty member has been successful in establishing good working relationships with staff in the clinical area and designing exciting learning experiences for students, that information could be shared with other faculty to help them do the same things in their agencies (or maybe new agencies need to be sought if the current ones are "too far gone"). When another faculty member develops some rather creative approaches to teaching certain areas of content, she could be asked to share those with her colleagues. When yet another faculty member finds a way to combine classroom teaching, clinical teaching, research and publication efforts, other faculty could benefit from those experiences. If people shared their successes and rewards, the ultimate outcome would be a faculty that is more excited about what it's doing, a greater responsiveness to the needs of the students, and a better quality program. Who could possibly lose with such a winning combination?

If higher education, and nursing education in particular, are to remain credible in the eyes of the public, the very real issue of quality needs to be addressed. I think we, in nursing, have some very unique problems in this area; however, I also think we have many unique assets to deal with the quality issue. I'm convinced that with open dialogue, the kind of sharing that you and I do, and an adequate knowledge base (e.g., of how to use various teaching strategies), our fine tradition of quality education in nursing can be continued. We shouldn't settle for mediocrity in our educational programs just as we shouldn't settle for it in the care we provide to clients.

I know you are not the type to accept mediocrity in yourself and that despite the very normal "down days," you strive for excellence. I *know* that about you. And you can be—and I am sure *are*—a role model to your colleagues in this area. Just remember . . . you can't control what other people do. You can only try to influence it. You can take comfort in knowing you are providing the best quality of education you can, given the constraints (of time, resources, etc.) put upon you. These efforts will be appreciated by your students and perhaps eventually by your faculty colleagues. *You'll* know that you have been working to meet the students' needs, not your own (at least most of the time), and that's what's most important. It's not an easy battle to fight, but as the saying goes, "Somebody's got to do it." Why not you?! Let me know how it goes.

7

Implementing the Curriculum Model: Negotiating Student Learning Experiences

In light of the many questions raised recently about higher education, educators from all disciplines are challenged to rethink what students are taught and the way knowledge is imparted (Gray, 1984). Much has been written about developing thinking skills of students. Criticisms leveled by those internal and external to the academic arena have suggested that students lack the skills needed to enter the work force with more than merely a set of technical capabilities. Scandals on Wall Street, within the ranks of the federal government, and in the religious community headline newspapers daily. Some sociopolitical analysts have suggested that the problems inherent in the ongoing corruption are related to the lack of and disregard for human beings. Focus on what "I" need to exist supersedes what is best for greater humankind.

With these thoughts in mind, the nurse educator of today is challenged to develop in students an ability to think, reason, and act for the purpose of meeting the needs of other individuals without an immediate "return on their investment." In addition to being capable of "caring" for their fellow human beings, neophyte nurses also must be technically competent. New graduate nurses must be able to think, act, and care in an environment that judges success by dollars saved. How a student is prepared to enter this arena can make all the difference in personal and professional outcomes. Herein lies the challenge for nurse educators.

USING THE CURRICULUM TO GUIDE LEARNING EXPERIENCES

Instructing students provides nurse educators with the opportunity to affect the future of nursing practice. How teachers structure the learning environment will greatly influence students' attitudes toward learning and the practice arena. Kramer's (1974) classic work helped educators appreciate that new graduates experience reality shock because the world of student learning and the world of nursing practice are very different. Practices that are insisted on in nursing school bear little or no resemblance to what is "real" in practice.

Since the time of Kramer's (1974) publication, nurse educators have worked even harder to provide more realistic learning experiences for students. Students are clear in their verbalizations about wanting to "do" what nurses do. For instance, undergraduates quickly observe that practicing nurses are able to complete their care planning activities in a short amount of time. Questions and comments surface repeatedly related to the requirement to carry out extensive care planning. Students appear to have limited appreciation for the time it takes to learn a new skill and the value of learning it completely before using shortcuts.

In an environment where students demand the opportunity to "do," faculty members are faced with the dilemma of creating learning situations that allow for the doing as well as the learning. This is not to suggest that the two are mutually exclusive, but rather to emphasize the importance of providing theoretical support for the practice skills used by nurses.

Keeping in mind students' perceptions of urgency relative to learning skills and the mission of collegiate institutions to develop thinkers, nurse educators have traditionally developed curricula to be responsive to both needs. These curricula reflect philosophies that contain the following (Yura, 1986):

> the faculty's belief about man generally and, more specifically, about man the learner, the teacher, the nurse practitioner, the consumer. The fac-

ulty's belief about nursing, about ... nursing education, about the present and the emerging roles of the graduate of the ... nursing program, about the teaching-learning process and about other beliefs designated as significant to faculty. (pp. 4–5)

Nursing education philosophies direct learning experiences. To support the philosophy, nursing education administration works with faculty to secure and develop resources to meet the needs levied by the nursing faculty beliefs that are identified in the philosophy.

If, for example, the nursing faculty in a particular college or university subscribes to the belief that the learner is a self directed adult in search of new knowledge, didactic and clinical learning opportunities would be developed to enable the learners to maximize their self direction. Lecture, for instance, would not be the most effective way of facilitating education of individuals who are cast as self directed learners. Thus, one could assume that the elements of the philosophy for this nursing department had been examined by the faculty and give direction to the information deemed essential for students, as well as the strategies used to impart it.

In addition to the philosophy, the National League for Nursing requires that the curriculum be logically organized (*Criteria for the Evaluation*, 1989, 1990). Many faculty groups have chosen to use an organizing framework to meet this criterion. The organizing framework is a less philosophical statement about the faculty's beliefs. Typically, the concepts of human beings, environment, nursing, and health are addressed. Pepper (1986) states, "I like to think of the organizational framework of the curriculum as the model that is structured from the major characteristics that provide the curriculum personality" (p. 12). It is the master plan that turns the philosophy into reality (Pepper, 1986).

The development of the philosophy leads to the development of the objectives of the program. From the philosophy and objectives, faculty members are able to develop the organizing framework. From the organizing framework flows the development of level and course objectives. One of the great difficulties with the implementation of a model of development as described earlier is the necessity to continue to be responsive to the needs of society and the health care system in particular. Philosophies, organizing frameworks, and objectives must be living, changing statements. The curriculum as a document must be responsive to the needs of faculty, students and the health care system.

A nursing model is used in some schools of nursing as the organizing framework. To demonstrate the utility of a nursing model in organizing a curriculum, an example of how Orem's (1985) conceptual model can be used will be offered.

The major premise of Orem's conceptual ideology is that individuals are interested in and directed toward their own care. Because from time to time individuals may be deficient in the prerequisite knowledge of how to care for themselves or for some reason may be unable to use the knowledge they do have, they may require the legitimate caregiver services that nurses provide. Within the framework of the nurse-patient relationship, nurses design nursing systems to meet health and illness needs that individuals are unable to provide for themselves.

Based on the information provided, if a school of nursing uses Orem (1985) to organize their curriculum, the philosophy, behavioral objectives, learning activities, and organization of content would reflect Orem's notions about nursing. For instance, approaches to student learning and patient care would reflect the belief that individuals are interested in caring for themselves. Theoretical information might be organized and presented using Orem's three types of nursing systems: wholly compensatory, partly compensatory, and supportive educative. These themes would guide faculty in deciding where specific theoretical content should be presented and which clinical settings would provide students with experiences relevant to the particular nursing system being studied.

The example offered earlier is cursory, at best, but it is intended to give the reader some idea of how a nursing model can be used to organize the curriculum. Individuals teaching in a program that uses a particular nursing model would do well to study the model and discuss fully how it guides the development and implementation of the curriculum.

LEARNING ACTIVITIES

The nursing literature abounds with suggestions for teaching strategies (de Tornyay & Thompson, 1987; Leach & Champion, 1989;

Margolius & Duffy, 1989; Spickerman, 1988). To maximize the use of particular teaching strategies, the nurse educator needs to ask about the purpose of the learning exercise, the information that is to be learned, and the structure of the group. In addition, instructors need to be cognizant of the philosophy, terminal behaviors, organizing framework, and level and course objectives of the program. With this information in mind, the nurse educator can decide which strategies will work best with specific content and particular learning groups.

Developing Critical Thinkers

Schön (1987) discusses the education of a reflective practitioner as a process of supporting self-discovery. He contends that few situations ever present themselves to professional practitioners with clear-cut answers. Schön suggests that in educating professional practitioners, educators must teach them to "reflect in action" (p. 26). Such statements are congruent with one of the goals of many baccalaureate programs, namely, to prepare critical thinkers. Although the logic and applicability of statements like those of Schön may seem obvious to some, there appears to be some questions about whether this is what new graduates have been taught when they enter the practice arena. Strategies for teaching and learning should support the development of critical thinkers.

Brookfield (1987) offers suggestions of how to facilitate the development of critical thinkers. Some of his suggestions include affirming the self-worth of critical thinkers, listening sensitively and attentively to what they have to say, demonstrating support for their efforts, reflecting and mirroring critical thinkers' ideas and actions, motivating them to think critically, helping critical thinkers to develop support networks, increasing awareness of how critical thinking is learned, modeling critical thinking, and being a critical teacher.

Support for critical thinking can be found in statements made by both the National League for Nursing (*Criteria for the Evaluation*, 1989, 1990) and the American Association of Colleges of Nursing (1986). Toliver (1988), Klaassens (1988) and Hahnemann (1986) offer suggestions on specific strategies that can be used to develop nursing students' abilities to think critically. Both Klaassens and Hahnemann discuss the use of writing as a way to develop critical thinking skills.

In a related article, Allen, Bowers, and Diekelmann (1989) suggest the development of writing skills to enhance learning. Writing to enhance critical thinking skills is just one example of the ways educators can use particular strategies to promote the development of specific skills.

Developing Creative Thinkers

In addition to promoting critical thinkers, many faculty members express a commitment to helping students develop their creative abilities. Clinical educators know that the practice world does not have "textbook" patients with clear-cut health problems. All too often the medical or nursing treatment prescribed for the patient falls short of being a perfect solution. Human beings and the problems they face are too complex for standardized answers. Frequently nurses must develop creative strategies to deal with problems that cannot be managed through routine, standard treatments.

In a discussion of creative thinkers, Brookfield (1987) tells us that creative thinkers generally defy convention. All too frequently educators must own up to the fact that students' acceptance of convention keeps classrooms running smoothly. Many times the teaching strategies employed, the evaluation mechanisms designed, and the content identified as essential are based solely on conventional wisdom about what is right. Egan (1986) states that creative thinkers have a predilection for nonconformity and are risk takers. Brookfield (1987, pp. 115–116) proposes that the following conceptualizations represent creative thinkers:

1. Creative thinkers reject standardized formats for problem solving.
2. They have interest in a wide range of related and divergent fields.
3. They can take multiple perspectives on a problem.
4. They view the world as relative and contextual rather than universal and absolute.
5. They frequently use trial-and-error methods in their experimentation with alternative approaches.
6. They have a future orientation; change is embraced optimistically as a valuable developmental possibility.
7. They have self-confidence and trust in their own judgment.

If the nurse educator uses these statements to guide the development of teaching and learning strategies, creative thinking can be supported in the classroom and the clinical setting. Although the creative student may be perceived as a difficult student, appreciation of particular learning needs of the creative thinker will enhance the learning environment for all those involved.

COLLABORATION AS A MEANS OF MAXIMIZING STUDENT POTENTIAL

Given the discussion of critical and creative thinkers, the nurse educator is challenged to develop practitioners who will be current the day they enter practice, as well as 10, 20, or 30 years later. With this thought in mind, the value and necessity of collaboration with those whose primary practice is in the clinical setting is suggested.

Nurses in clinical practice should be made part of curriculum development, revision, implementation, and evaluation. Individuals who work in the practice setting can inform nurse educators about the changes that occur on a regular basis. This is not to suggest that each time a new piece of equipment becomes available in a clinical setting that faculty should immediately add a laboratory lecture to discuss it. If practitioners advise nurse educators about curricular issues, the latter will remain informed about changes affecting the health care setting and thereby keep the curriculum relevant. For instance, if students are leaving the collegiate settings with a limited or inadequate knowledge base relative to nursing care of individuals with immunosuppressive problems, then this is certainly something that needs to be addressed in the curriculum. The issue that guides curriculum change and changes in teaching and learning strategies should not be a new drug or therapy for treating AIDS patients, but rather the principles that would guide the care of individuals who experience immunosuppression.

Principles, not technology, should guide curricular change. As the technology changes, the principles that guided the initial learning of particular skills will be useful in the further development and refinement of skills related to a new technology.

SUMMARY

This chapter has given an overview of the challenges that nurse educators face in implementing curriculum models. Specifically it has addressed the concerns relative to negotiating experiences for students that will enhance their critical and creative thinking abilities. Also suggested is the importance of including practitioners as advisers for curriculum development and revision in an effort to inform nurse educators of the changes that will affect graduates entering the practice arena.

REFERENCES

Allen, D. G., Bowers, B., & Diekelmann, N. (1989). Writing to learn: A reconceptualization of thinking and writing in the nursing curriculum. *Journal of Nursing Education, 28*(1), 6–11.

American Association of Colleges of Nursing. (1986). *Essentials of college and university education for professional nursing.* Washington, DC: American Association of Colleges of Nursing.

Brookfield, S. D. (1987). *Developing critical thinkers.* San Francisco: Jossey-Bass.

Criteria for the evaluation of associate degree programs in nursing (7th ed.). (1990). New York: National League for Nursing.

Criteria for the evaluation of baccalaureate and higher degree programs in nursing (6th ed.). (1989). New York: National League for Nursing.

de Tornyay, R., & Thompson, M. A. (1987). *Strategies for teaching nursing* (3rd ed.). New York: Wiley.

Egan, G. (1986). *The skilled helper: A systematic approach to effective helping* (3rd ed.). Monterey, CA: Brooks-Cole.

Gray, J. G. (1984). *Re-thinking American education* (2nd ed.). Middletown, CT: Wesleyan University Press.

Hahnemann, B. K. (1986). Journal writing: A key to promoting critical thinking in nursing students. *Journal of Nursing Education, 25*(5), 213–215.

Klaassens, E. L. (1988). Improving teaching for thinking. *Nurse Educator, 13*(6), 15–19.

Kramer, M. (1974). *Reality shock: Why nurses are leaving.* St. Louis: Mosby.

Leach, A., & Champion, V. (1989). Research teaching strategies. *Nurse Educator, 14*(1), 5.

Margolius, F. R., & Duffy, M. M. (1989). Promoting creativity: The use of student projects. *Nurse Educator, 14*(2), 32–35.

Orem, D. E. (1985). *Nursing: Concepts of practice* (3rd ed.). New York: McGraw-Hill.

Pepper, J. M. (1986). The essential ingredient in curriculum design: The organizing framework. In E. A. Pennington (Ed.), *Curriculum revisited: An update of curriculum design* (pp. 11–24). New York: National League for Nursing.

Schön, D. A. (1987). *Educating the reflective practitioner*. San Francisco: Jossey-Bass.

Spickerman, S. (1988). Enhancing the socialization process. *Nurse Educator, 13*(6), 10–13.

Toliver, J. C. (1988). Inductive reasoning; Critical thinking skills for clinical competence. *Clinical Nurse Specialist, 2*(4), 174–179.

Yura, H. (1986). Curriculum development process. In National League for Nursing, *Faculty-curriculum development: Curriculum design by nursing faculty* (pp. 3–10). New York: National League for Nursing.

8

Education and Service: Interdependent Players in Nursing

The process of educating nursing students for beginning professional roles is a complex, multifaceted one that will be successful only with the cooperation and collaboration among many players. If the educational experience is to contribute to the total development of students and provide them with the knowledge, skills, and values necessary to practice professional nursing now and in the future, it must be a joint enterprise in which nurse educators, faculty in other disciplines, students themselves, consumers, and nurses in clinical agencies must participate.

Nurses in education and those in the service setting must recognize that if they work together, rather than working "at odds" with each other, the graduates of educational programs will be better prepared to assume responsible professional positions. Although "collaboration between nursing education and nursing service is a concept with which few take exception philosophically" (Styles, 1985, p. 175), and although many in our field have expressed concern about "the negative consequences of fragmentation and divisiveness" (Styles, 1985, p 175), unity between these two groups of nurses is far from being achieved.

Perhaps this lack of unity is a reflection of the tumultuous history of nursing education-service relationships, and perhaps it relates to a lack of knowledge about how to enhance collaboration. Both of these possible causes are important to explore because nursing can no longer afford to allow such discontinuity to persist. Nursing's future in the educational arena, the service setting, and the health care delivery system in general will be influenced by the interdependence of nursing education and nursing service; that relationship must be recognized, valued, and enhanced.

HISTORICAL BACKGROUND

In the early days of the profession, nursing education and service were intimately intertwined. The origins of the profession are deeply embedded in service agencies, and for a century the control of education was in hospitals.

Nursing's early system of education was primarily an apprenticeship-type one, with the neophyte learning from the practicing nurse. The reality of the day-to-day practice world was the classroom, the staff nurse was, in large part, the teacher, and the content that the neophyte learned was whatever he or she "needed to know to get through the day." Education was clearly a subset of service, being subservient to service's need for cheap labor and staffing of unpopular shifts.

Almost since the profession's very beginnings, however, nurse leaders decried the apprenticeship system and called for the education of nurses to occur in institutions of higher learning where (a) students' needs to learn would take priority over the hospital's need for staff; (b) students would not be exploited; (c) the education of nurses would be controlled by academics, as was true in other disciplines; and (d) new members of the profession could be instilled with a visionary idealism of what could be, as well as with a picture of what is. A formalized position by nursing on this concept did not occur until the American Nurses' Association's *Position Paper* (1965), but the calls for it began before the turn of this century and have been documented time and again since then.

The original model in which education and service were essentially one entity certainly had many strengths. Several social, political, economic, and professional developments have occurred to move nursing away from such a model, however.

Wagner (1980) asserted that one of the major changes that served to swing the pendulum in another direction was the move of education out of hospitals. The result of this, she asserted, was defensiveness on the part of both education and service, and battles over territory, status, and power.

The second major change that Wagner (1980) cited as having had a significant impact on the nature of the relationship between nursing education and nursing service was the development and eventual evolution of associate degree programs. When the associate degree model was originally proposed in the 1950s, it was clearly stated that the focus of such programs was to prepare a technical nurse with a more limited scope of practice. The limits to that practice were defined, and graduates of such programs were not intended to be identical to or assume the same responsibilities as graduates of other programs.

Unfortunately, either this initial intent was not heard, or it was ignored. Licensing examinations were not developed for this technical level of practice, and employers—rightfully so—expected these licensed registered nurses (RNs) to function as other licensed RNs did. Given the original intent of associate degree programs, these early graduates may not have been as skilled or capable as graduates of other programs, and employers were dissatisfied, complaining that education "was not doing its job." Although the purpose of this discussion is not to debate the value of associate degree education in nursing, it is important to realize that the original intent of those programs was lost somehow, and a result was the growing dissatisfaction between nursing education and nursing service.

Changes in baccalaureate education also contributed to this growing dissatisfaction. In response to existing and projected changes in educational patterns and in health care, collegiate programs began to move away from the traditional type of educational structures and experiences.

As nurses looked toward new roles and toward increasing the professional dimensions of their practice, collegiate programs responded. No longer was it appropriate for students to have all of their clinical experiences in hospitals. Nurses were looking to provide care to well individuals as well as sick ones, to families as well as individuals, and to communities. They were concerned about developing the body of nursing knowledge, about conducting and using nursing research, and about developing and using theory as a basis for practice. They were also establishing practices in schools, clinics, health maintenance organizations, correctional facilities, and independent offices, as well as in hospitals.

If the educational institution was to fulfill its mission of preparing individuals for tomorrow as well as for today, it had to provide a variety of opportunities for students to experience such roles, settings, and responsibilities. As a result, students had less experience in the traditional hospital setting and, when they were there, they focused less on technologies, routines, and procedures.

The service setting's values and those of the educational institution had become very different. Our accumulated habits and traditions no longer worked, and the pendulum had swung to the opposite extreme where education and service were miles apart—geographically, philosophically, and in other ways.

STATE OF THE ART

Peters (1980) said that the gap between education and service is the *real* split in nursing. She urged that "educators should get out of their 'ivory tower[s]' and clinical practitioners out of the 'trenches' to solve the real crisis in nursing—[namely], their constant opposition" (p. 107).

Today, nursing service and nursing education are isolated in many ways. Each lives in its own world, and although they coexist, their connectedness is limited. Each world has its own goals and agendas and operates out of a different frame of reference, the latter of which influences how an organization or a collective behaves.

The "walls" created over the years between nursing education and nursing practice are real. They can be understood, however; and, if they can be understood, then they can be managed and broken down. The "walls" between these two arenas of nursing practice may be thought of as falling into several categories.

Misunderstanding

Nurses in education and service do not fully understand each other's work world, goals, constraints, values, possibilities, needs, and so on. This results in a lack of trust in each other and a lack of collegiality.

Miscommunication

Nurses in education and service miscommunicate or fail to communicate altogether concerning their purposes, strengths, accomplishments, problems, needs, and so forth. They go to separate conferences, read separate journals, belong to separate interest groups, and, in essence, are isolated from one another, failing to share and failing to collaborate.

Inadequate or Inappropriate Coping Mechanisms

Nurse educators and nursing service administrators are facing fiscal crises and reduction or elimination of federal and other kinds of support, and they operate in highly stressful situations. In dealing with these crises nurses often blame one another, engage in internal rivalry, and attach negative labels to one another, instead of pooling the resources available to deal with issues that affect all (e.g., the recruitment of adequate numbers of qualified individuals).

Socialization and Language

Nurses are socialized, throughout much of their nursing education (if not their whole lives), to look at problems, what's wrong, the negative, the diagnosis, or the disease. Yes, they learn that the next step after identifying the problem is to figure out what to do about it, but the initial orientation is on the negative instead of the positive; De Feo (1987, p. 270) referred to this phenomenon as "the hunt for the really bad nurse." With such an orientation ingrained in them, nurses may find it too easy to focus on each other's limitations and differences rather than on each other's strengths and commonalities.

Lack of Knowledge

Finally, a "wall" between nursing education and nursing service may be related to a lack of knowledge of how to work together. Nurses have experienced so many problems for so long that they may not know how to begin to manage them.

APPROACHES TO COLLABORATION

Throughout the years, individual nurses in practice and individual nursing faculty members have made efforts to break down the walls and bridge the real or potential gaps between these two groups, and they have been most successful. In such instances, students have had very positive learning experiences, nursing staff members have been challenged, patients have received excellent care, and the individuals involved in planning such experiences have been rewarded.

In addition, many recent reports of new collaborative efforts between nursing education and service have been shared. Service settings are offering scholarships to attract individuals to enter and remain in nursing education programs. Educational programs are redesigning undergraduate and graduate program content and structures to accommodate RNs who need or want to continue to work while they go to school. Hospitals are expanding extern, intern, preceptor, and mentor programs to meet the needs of new nurses, and nursing faculty members are participating in the implementation of such programs. These are but a few examples of collaborative efforts, but they demonstrate the interdependence of nursing education and nursing service.

Such collaboration is critical if nursing students are to have positive, rewarding learning experiences and be enthusiastic about nursing. Nurse educators play a large part in ensuring such success.

One of the first ways to provide for good learning experiences is to select clinical agencies carefully (Bevil & Gross, 1981). Each nursing program should develop a list of criteria that is used when clinical agencies and specific clinical units are selected for student affiliations. Among such criteria, faculty may want to consider the following: the accreditation-approval status of the agency, the adequacy of staffing (in terms of numbers, qualifications, and capabilities), the number and type of patients available, the extent to which specific course objectives can be met, the attitudes of the nursing staff toward students (particularly students from the type of program in which one teaches), and the expressed willingness of the staff to work with the faculty member and students.

Once the agency and specific clinical units are selected, the faculty and unit coordinator as well as the department chair or dean and the nursing director of the agency should be aware of the aspects of the contract or letter of agreement that has been signed. (A copy of this contract usually is on file in the office of the nursing dean or department chair, and the agency's director of nursing or clinical affiliations coordinator.) For example, the contract may specify that conference space will be provided for students and faculty on the unit; however, if unit coordinators are not aware of this detail and had previously been directed to use conference space only for their own staff, they may hesitate to allot the space, faculty members may feel unsupported in their efforts, and the relationship will be strained. Thus, all parties affected should be well aware of what has and has not been agreed on in the signed contract.

Faculty members must take responsibility for communicating the students' learning objectives and their status in the program (i.e., graduating seniors or sophomores in their first clinical experience) to everyone involved in the learning experience—the agency's affiliations coordinator, the unit coordinator or head nurse, and the individual staff on the unit. Such communications should occur well in advance of the learning experience, again just before it begins, and all through it; it may take the form of letters that are accompanied by a curriculum plan and a course syllabus, telephone calls, one-to-one meetings, or attendance at staff meetings. It is essential that the staff on the unit knows (a) the level of the students who will be practicing on the unit, (b) the specific learning objectives, and (c) what students can and cannot do; otherwise, staff may have expectations that are far beyond or far below what they could be.

Nursing faculty members may do well to reflect on the extent to which they involve staff in the students' learning experiences. Although the objectives for the experience are designed by the entire faculty, via the curriculum committee, and the responsibility for evaluating students rests with the faculty member, there is no reason why staff nurses cannot be an integral part of the learning experience. Students should feel free to approach staff nurses with questions or with information about patients' conditions; staff should be invited to explain and demonstrate things to students.

Faculty members who convey an attitude of "come to me, not the staff" concerning questions are devaluing what the staff nurses know and can do, failing to help students develop the collegial interactions that will be critical to their practice after graduating, and causing unnecessary stress for themselves. It would be inappropriate and irresponsible for a faculty member to disengage totally from the students' activities on the unit, expecting the staff nurses to "do it all." A healthy balance of these two approaches, however, would greatly benefit the students, the staff, the patients, and the faculty member.

One of the criticisms often leveled at nursing faculty in the clinical area is that they are not clinically expert, and faculty may need to deal with such a "charge." This can be done by practicing as a staff nurse before the semester begins, by helping students and staff solve clinical problems, and by explaining the difference between clinical expertise and clinical competence. There would seem to be no excuse for faculty who are not clinically *competent* in the area in which they are teaching students. Clinical *expertise*, however, may not be possible to attain by anyone except those who deal with selected problems and situations on a continuous basis.

The primary role of nursing faculty members is that of teacher, not clinician; a secondary role, often mandated for faculty in senior colleges and universities, is that of researcher-scholar, not clinician. Thus, nursing faculty members should be expected to be expert teachers and scholars (or provide extensive service at the junior college level), but not expert clinicians. When faculty and staff recognize this reality, it often makes it easier for them to draw on each other's strengths and to collaborate more effectively.

In enhancing relationships between education and service, faculty members may want to reconsider some practices that have, perhaps, become tradition. For example, if they find that staff has gone ahead and done some procedures or patient teaching without waiting for the students to be involved, the faculty member may want to reexamine whether beginning the clinical day at 8 a.m. with a 1-hour preconference (which keeps the students off the units until 9 a.m. when the day shift started at 7 a.m.) is the best arrangement. Could students begin their clinical day at 7 a.m.? Could they report at 8 a.m. and have a very brief preconference? Could preconferencing be done on a one-to-one basis with each student? Or could students report to the unit, do some basic interventions with their patients (e.g., vital signs and medications), and then report for a preconference at 9 a.m.? Arguments could be made for each of these alternatives, and no one option is always the best under all circumstances. Thus, the faculty member, perhaps in collaboration with the unit coordinator, could implement a different approach to this problem and resolve it to the satisfaction of everyone.

There are many other approaches to promoting the interdependence of nursing education and nursing service in which nursing faculty may be involved. Aydelotte (1985) classified these approaches to "conjoining nursing education and practice" (p. 288) as relating to changes in organizational structures, collaborative financing of nursing education, faculty practice, clinical experiences for students, and the transition of new graduates into practice roles.

Specific activities for collaboration have included the following: joint appointments to both agencies (Kuhn, 1982), joint practice models (Blazeck, Selekman, Timpe, & Wolf, 1982; Cochran et al., 1989; Ingber & Peddicord, 1989; Nayer, 1980; Westcot, 1981); collaborative research efforts (Engstrom, 1984); and shared projects (e.g., orientation of new staff) (Schwab & Simmons, 1989; Werner, 1980). Schools of nursing and clinical agencies also may wish to share newsletters and other publications or communications, serve on each other's committees, and engage in role exchange experiences that have proved valuable to some groups (Eschbach, 1983).

Work-study or cooperative education arrangements (Huckstadt, 1981) may be workable models between some institutions, as may be graduate nurse transition programs (Borovies & Newman, 1981). Schools and clinical agencies may find it beneficial to use staff nurses as clinical teachers (Clark, 1981), establish partnerships (Barrell & Hamric, 1986; Sorensen, Gassman, & Walters, 1984), institute three-way (student-staff-teacher) conferences (Fishel, 1982), and initiate or strengthen preceptor-internship programs (Donius, 1988; Friesen & Conahan, 1980; May, 1980; Walters, 1981). Both groups also might benefit from developing publication support groups or joint publication activities (Hale & Pruitt, 1989); developing orientation manuals for students, faculty, and staff (Fortune & Torres, 1983); or issuing joint position statements and testimony on relevant nursing and health care issues.

In addition, offering guest lectures or continuing education programs in each other's institutions; establishing interinstitutional interdisciplinary management teams (Fitzpatrick & Behrman, 1985); instituting scholar-in-residence or clinician-in-residence programs; sharing physical resources (e. g., classrooms, audiovisual materials, computer hardware, and software); and even changing the curriculum so it is more responsive to current demands, trends, and expectations (Dexter & Laidig, 1980) also may be helpful. Finally, increasing opportunities for social exchange and communication (e.g., a welcome coffeehouse for students and faculty at the agency, or a back-to-school social at the university to which agency staff is invited), and scheduling regular meetings for planning and problem solving on an ongoing basis are strategies that could enhance and strengthen the relationship between nursing education and nursing service.

SUMMARY

Despite the fact that each arena has different reward systems, different values, different governance structures, and different expectations for its members, nurses in education and those in practice share common concerns about quality education, quality patient care, and the viability of our profession. Efforts such as those cited here serve to recognize the differences and to emphasize the commonalities.

As Billie (1986) warned, "Unless nursing service and education work toward a symbiotic relationship, the gaps between them will increase and each will experience increased difficulties" (p. 1). Such symbiotic relationships need to be promoted by schools with all the clinical facilities with which they affiliate for student learning experiences. Likewise, service agencies need to foster such relationships with all the schools that affiliate at their facilities. Thus, an "us" rather than a "we-they" (Walker, 1984) perspective and approach will be most beneficial to all players in this interdependent "game."

According to Walker (1985), to build bridges between nursing education and nursing service, a commitment to a larger purpose and the broader profession, a willingness to accept responsibility for helping each other, realistic expectations of one another, and flexibility are needed. All this requires maturity and mutual respect.

"After a period of denying [our common] roots, we are now beginning to see the benefits of mutual support" (Joel, 1985, p. 221). Such benefits of education-service collaboration include the following: the increased power of nursing to shape the future, better care for the public, and a better public understanding of nursing. It can also result in an improved image and enhanced visibility of nursing and an increased respect and support for the discipline.

Collaboration between nursing education and service also can yield decreased costs of recruitment, orientation and on-the-job training, an exemplary learning climate for students and staff, and decreased job changes, burnout, apathy, and withdrawal from nursing. In addition, more sophisticated and meaningful research, with a greater chance of research findings being used to guide practice, an expansion of nursing's knowledge base, and significant innovations in practice and education are potential outcomes.

Finally, interdependent efforts can yield added resources and opportunities for growth, an improved use of material and human resources, and the increased recognition by nurses of their responsibility—not only for their individual practice, but for the improvement of the profession as a whole through collegial sharing. All of this will recognize and promote the clinical expertise of staff nurses and demonstrate to neophyte nurses that intradisciplinary collaboration is vital and beneficial to their own growth and to that of the profession as a whole.

Nurse educators are concerned about the profession and, particulary, about providing excellent learning experiences for students. As such, they must work to merge the best of both worlds—education and service.

> If we fail to join forces, if we go our separate competitive ways duplicating our efforts, if we collide rather than collaborate, we will dissipate our limited finances and valuable time, energy, and other resources. And we will continually undermine our mission, as well as our position in society. (Walker, 1984, p. 10)

It seems nursing can ill afford—for nurses themselves, the profession as a whole, and the students who are hoping to become colleagues—to fail to join forces.

REFERENCES

American Nurses' Association. (1965). *Educational preparation for nurse practitioners and assistants to nurses: A position paper*. New York: Author.

Aydelotte, M. K. (1985). Approaches to conjoining nursing education and practice. In J. C. McCloskey & H. K. Grace (Eds.), *Current issues in nursing* (2nd ed.) (pp. 288–313). Boston: Blackwell Scientific Publications.

Barrell, L. M., & Hamric, A. B. (1986). Education and service: A collaborative model to improve patient care. *Nursing & Health Care, 7*(9), 497–503.

Bevil, C. W., & Gross, L. C. (1981). Assessing the adequacy of clinical learning settings. *Nursing Outlook, 29*(11), 658–661.

Billie, D. A. (1986). Service and education: Time for symbiosis [Editorial]. *Journal of Nursing Education, 25*(1), 1.

Blazeck, A. M., Selekman, J., Timpe, M., & Wolf, Z. (1982). Unification: Nursing education and nursing practice. *Nursing & Health Care, 3*(1), 18–24.

Borovies, D. L., & Newman, N. A. (1981). Graduate nursing transition programs. *American Journal of Nursing, 81*(10), 1832–1835.

Clark, M. D. (1981). Staff nurses as clinical teachers. *American Journal of Nursing, 81*(2), 314–319.

Cochran, L. L., Ambutas, S. A., Buckley, J. K., D'Arco, S. H., Donovan, M. I., Fruth, R. M., Monico, L. U., & Scherubel, J. C. (1989). The unification model: A collaborative effort. *Nursing Connections, 2*(1), 5–17.

De Feo, D. (1987). The search for the really bad nurse. *American Journal of Nursing, 87*(2), 270.

Dexter, P. A., & Laidig, J. (1980). Breaking the education/service barrier. *Nursing Outlook, 28*(3), 179–182.

Donius, M. A. (1988). The Columbia precepting program: Building a bridge with clinical faculty. *Journal of Professional Nursing, 4*(1), 17–22.

Engstrom, J. L. (1984). University, agency, and collaborative models for nursing research: An overview. *Image: The Journal of Nursing Scholarship, 16*(3), 76–79.

Eschbach, D. (1983). Role exchange: An exciting experiment. *Nursing Outlook, 31*(3), 164–167.

Fishel, A. H. (1982). The three-way conference: Nursing student, nurse supervisor, and nurse educator. *Journal of Nursing Education, 20*(6), 18–23.

Fitzpatrick, J. J., & Behrman, R. E. (1985). The university and the hospital: Old friends, new allies. *Nursing & Health Care, 6*(7), 383–384.

Fortune, M., & Torres, C. S. (1983). Service-education collaboration in a community health agency. *Nursing & Health Care, 4*(8), 448–449.

Friesen, L., & Conahan, B. J. (1980). A clinical preceptor program: Strategy for new graduate orientation. *Journal of Nursing Administration, 10*(4), 18–23.

Hale, S. L., & Pruitt, R. H. (1989). Enhancing publication success. *Nursing Connections, 2*(1), 59–61.

Huckstadt, A. A. (1981). Work/study: A bridge to practice. *American Journal of Nursing, 81*(4), 726–727.

Ingber, I., & Peddicord, K. (1989). The dyad model of nursing practice. *Nursing Connections, 2*(1), 21–30.

Joel, L. (1985). The Rutgers experience: One perspective on service-education collaboration. *Nursing Outlook, 33*(6), 220–224.

Kuhn, J. A. (1982). An experiment with a joint appointment. *American Journal of Nursing, 82*(10), 1570–1571.

May, L. (1980). Clinical preceptors for new nurses. *American Journal of Nursing, 80*(10), 1824–1826.

Nayer, D. (1980). Unification: Bringing nursing service and nursing education together. *American Journal of Nursing, 80*(6), 1110–1114.

Peters, V. J. (1980). "Ivory tower" vs. practice: The real split in nursing [Sound off!]. *RN, 43*(9), 107–108, 110.

Schwab, T., & Simmons, R. (1989). Collaboration in action. *Nursing Connections, 2*(1), 35–42.

Sorenson, G., Gassman, A., & Walters, M. (1984). An experiment in a working relationship between nursing education and nursing service. *Journal of Nursing Education, 23*(2), 81–83.

Styles, M. M. (1985). Collaboration: Essential to public acceptance [Editorial]. *Nursing & Health Care, 6*(4), 175.

Wagner, D. L. (1980). Nursing administrator's assessment of nursing education. *Nursing Outlook, 28*(9), 557–561.

Walker, D. D. (1984). Beyond "we/they." *Stanford Nurse, 6*(3), 10.

Walker, D. D. (1985). Nursing education and service: The payoffs of partnership. *Nursing & Health Care, 6*(4), 189–191.

Walters, C. R. (1981). Using staff preceptors in a senior experience. *Nursing Outlook, 29*(4), 245–247.

Werner, J. (1980). Joint endeavors: The way to bring service and education together. *Nursing Outlook, 28*(9), 546–550.

Westcot, L. B. (1981). Nursing education and nursing service: A collaborative model. *Nursing & Health Care, 2*(7), 376–379.

9

Evaluation of Students: A Major Faculty Responsibility

Along with the responsibility for teaching is the concomitant duty to evaluate what students learn. The accountability required for evaluation makes some educators uncomfortable, particularly when the outcome of the evaluation process may affect the student's future in a deleterious way. To develop a positive outlook on the evaluation process, the nurse educator should learn as much as possible about the process to promote a positive outcome for the learner as well as for the teacher.

The goal of evaluation is to give learners a measure of expected performance behavior. The evaluation tells learners how successfully they have met particular objectives.

Most students and educators would agree that when learning occurs, it does so with a goal in mind. For instance, if a student wishes to learn to play the piano, at some point the ability to accomplish this activity will be measured against a predefined standard. For piano students, the standard might be being able to play "Twinkle Twinkle Little Star" without making errors. To meet the objective of playing the piece without a mistake, students will need to learn how to move their fingers on the keyboard, read music, and play the piece with "style." As trite as this example may seem, most learning occurs with a particular outcome in mind. In addition to the outcome is a standard that is used to develop the outcome.

For a nursing student interested in learning to insert a foley catheter, the outcome may be successful insertion of the catheter. The standards for performance can be manifold. The student may wish to complete the insertion in a fashion that mimics that of a professional nurse, to complete the task without needing guidance from the faculty member, or to complete the insertion without hurting the patient. Students will rate themselves based on the predetermined standard.

In addition to the student's standard, however, is the professional standard. In teaching the professional standard, faculty members have the responsibility to evaluate the degree to which the student measures up to a set of predefined criteria and expectations. Although the standard against which the student's performance is measured can be made objective, the evaluation of the degree to which one meets the standard is far less so. According to Litwack, Linc, & Bower (1985), evaluation "is the process of appraising the meaning of the data gathered through one or more measurements" (p. 5). It is precisely the attachment of meaning that may leave educators feeling uncomfortable about the evaluation process.

Evaluation of any activity should be a process that results in a decision on how the learner has met a standard. The outcomes or standards that will be used to evaluate students must be known to them before the evaluation. In addition, students must have time to develop the necessary cognitive or psychomotor skills on which they will be evaluated. This raises several questions for the educator. One that is repeatedly offered by nurse educators in relation to evaluation in the clinical area is: At what point does learning end and evaluation begin? Another question frequently asked is: Should I measure the students against each other's performance or against specific criteria? A third question that occasionally arises in faculty meetings is: Am I measuring students on what they have learned or on what is tested on the licensing exam? All three of these questions are commonly heard and deserve further discussion.

SUMMATIVE AND FORMATIVE EVALUATION

The question of when to evaluate plagues many educators. Whether designing a class outline or observing students in the clinical setting, the nurse educator is forced to determine at what points in time demonstration of competence in the content area is necessary. Regardless of the setting, the evaluation point becomes a value judgment for the teacher. Typically, when defining classroom testing times, there is usually a logical break in content, such as the end of a unit in the textbook. The point for evaluation in the clinical setting is less clear. Generally, schools of nursing use the midpoint and the end of a clinical rotation as evaluation times. Having multiple evaluation points provides the learner with regular feedback on performance. This type of evaluation is referred to as formative evaluation. According to Litwack, Linc, & Bower (1985), "Formative evaluation usually involves the continual gathering of evaluative data throughout a learning experience" (p. 8).

Another type of evaluation that typically uses the data collected during formative evaluation is summative evaluation. Summative evaluation is an end-of-an-experience evaluation, such as a final examination. Both types of evaluation are valuable to both the student and the educator. Formative evaluation assists students in gauging their progress toward predefined outcomes. Summative evaluation ultimately measures the degree to which the student has met the expectations of a learning experience.

OVERVIEW OF EVALUATION MEASURES

Before moving on to the other two frequently asked questions, discussion of some of the types of evaluation measures used might be helpful. Generally nursing educators evaluate students in two areas: theoretical and clinical. Theoretical evaluation addresses the material that students learn in relation to the theory portion of the course, that is, classroom learning. Clinical evaluation focuses on the knowledge and skills the student is required to develop to care for patients.

Testing students' learning of theoretical material is less subjective and more controllable than measuring their clinical learning. Nurse educators, for the most part, measure theoretical knowledge through the use of objective pencil and paper tests. Clinical knowledge is most often measured in the clinical setting where few controls are possible. Clinical evaluation, therefore, can be very subjective. Nurse educators in the clinical setting use their observations of student behavior to decide what is and is not acceptable performance. Evaluation of psycho-motor skills occurs most often in the clinical setting or in a simulation laboratory setting. In the simulated laboratory controls are available that provide for an objective assessment of the students' abilities. Un-like the simulated laboratory, however, the clinical setting is an unpre-dictable place where extraneous problems arise that can leave the measurement of a particular skill or set of skills unevaluated.

Multiple-Choice Test Construction

The most commonly used measurement of theoretical knowledge is the pencil-and-paper test. Several ways are available to use this mea-surement strategy. The most popular one in prelicensure programs is the multiple-choice test. This type of test has the advantage of being versatile and adaptable across several content areas. Multiple-choice examination is a preferred testing approach among many nursing edu-cators because of its use in the NCLEX examination.

One of the issues that arises frequently in the development of multiple-choice tests is the reliability and validity of the items. Addi-tionally, the leveling and quality of test items concern test developers.

Examination Blueprint

Regarding leveling of test items, it is essential that test writers de-velop a blueprint for examination development. The purpose of a blueprint is to ensure that objectives are met, all pertinent informa-tion is covered, and more than the recall of facts is addressed. Frisbie (1983) offers that the use of a test blueprint "channels the thinking of the test developer to consider different levels of intellectual demand within each content area" (p. 229). Bloom's (1956) taxonomy is useful for directing test item construction as it relates to leveling of the items. Bloom's cognitive taxonomy includes the general categories of knowledge, comprehension, application, analysis, synthesis, and evalu-ation. Measurement in the affective domain according to Krathwohl, Bloom, and Masia (1964) includes receiving, responding, valuing, or-ganizing and characterizing of a value or value complex. For further discussion of these categories, the reader is referred to Krathwohl, Bloom, and Masia (1964).

Table 9.1. Test Blueprint For Multiple-Choice Nursing Process Examination (50 Items)

Taxonomy level	Content areas/objectives			
	Assessment	Planning	Intervention	Evaluation
Knowledge	3	3	3	2
Comprehension	3	3	3	3
Application	3	3	3	3
Analysis	2	1	2	2
Synthesis	0	0	0	0
Evaluation	2	2	2	2

A useful way to develop a blueprint is to review the objectives and content to be tested, outline the information that is important to the evaluation of it, and then write the items according to a test blueprint. In the example provided in Table 9.1 the reader is directed to the synthesis section of the blueprint. As can be seen, no items appear in this section. According to Frisbie (1983), objective tests are not well suited to the testing of analysis, synthesis, and evaluation. Similarly, it is difficult to use multiple-choice examinations to evaluate the affective domain. Short-answer or essay examinations, class papers, or projects would provide the students with the opportunity to demonstrate their abilities in these areas. With this in mind, in addition to multiple-choice items, short-answer or essay questions may need to be added to assure that all domains are included.

Validity

After defining the content to be tested and leveling the questions, the next step is to ensure the validity of the examination. According to Gronlund (1981). "validity refers to the *results* of a test or evaluation instrument for a given group of individuals, *not* the instrument itself" (p. 66). Content validity is the commonest type of validity measure used by nurse educators in the development of classroom tests. Achieving satisfactory content validity occurs by noting whether the test items functioned as they were intended. To strengthen the test items and increase the likelihood that they function as intended, Huben-Stanton (1983, p. 339) recommends the following:

1. The question or statement (stem) should be stated so that only a specific response is justifiable.
2. Choices or alternative responses to the individual multiple-choice items should be brief, accurate, occur at the end of the stem, and be approximately all the same length.
3. All the possible responses to a particular question should be grammatically consistent with the phraseology of the related stem.
4. Negatively stated or ambiguous items should always be avoided.
5. All possible responses to a particular item should be plausible.
6. To ensure a reasonable degree of difficulty of a particular multiple-choice item at least four alternative responses are necessary.
7. Each multiple-choice item should contain an independent problem that gives no clue to the answers of the remaining multiple-choice items on the test.

Reliability

Reliability of multiple choice tests is another area of concern for test writers. The American Psychological Association (1985) defines reliability in testing as the "degree to which scores are free from errors of measurement" (p. 19). Reliability then refers "to the results obtained with an evaluation instrument and not to the instrument itself" (Gronlund, 1981, p. 94). According to Flynn and Reese (1988) errors arise from "item sampling, anxiety, fear, effort, guessing, and other factors that affect the test taker's performance" (p. 62). Given these sources of error, it is impossible to develop a test that is completely free of errors; however, it is the responsibility of the test developer to make the test as free from errors as possible. To determine the reliability of a particular test, statistical analysis will be necessary. Some of the methods that can be used to measure the reliability of the examination results include test-retest, equivalent forms, split-half, and Kuder-Richardson. The reader is directed to measurement texts (Anastasi, 1982;Gronlund, 1981) for a full discussion of these methods.

Item Difficulty and Discrimination Power

In addition to reliability and validity measures, test developers are frequently interested in the difficulty of the items in the examination and the discrimination index. Item difficulty describes the percentage of students who marked an item correctly and gives the test writer an indication of how difficult an item is. According to Flynn and Reese (1988), "A test with moderate difficulty, i.e., one in which 50% to 80% of the class answered the items correctly, can be used to maximally differentiate among students" (p. 63).

Gronlund (1981) states that the discrimination index or power "refers to the degree to which it discriminate between pupils with high and low achievement" (p. 259). This computation helps the educator to determine whether the items as written discriminate between the students who are well prepared or who understand the material being tested and those who are not. The following paragraphs give examples of how to calculate item difficulty and item discrimination.

A class of 50 students has taken a 100-item examination. First, place all the examinations in graded order (i.e., 100, 97, 95, 95, 92, etc.). Next, take the top 14 examinations (approximately 27%) and the lower 14 examinations. The other 22 examinations will not be used for the analysis, so put them aside. In situations in which fewer than 25 students have taken an examination, divide the 25 in half and use the entire group for the analysis.

For each test item, tabulate the response choice made by students in the upper and lower groups (Table 9.2).

Table 9.2. Tabulation of Students' Response Choice

Students	Alternatives					Index	
	A	B	C[a]	D	Omit	Diff.[b]	Discr.[c]
Upper 14	0	2	12	0	0	.64	.43
Lower 14	2	6	6	0	0		

[a]Correct response. [b]Diff. = difficulty. [c]Discr. = discrimination.

To compute the *item difficulty,* the following formula is used:

$$\text{Item difficulty} = \frac{R}{T} \times 100$$

R = number of students who got the item right.
T = number of pupils who tried the item.

Using the data supplied from Table 9.2, the following represents the analysis.

$$\text{Item difficulty} = \frac{18}{28} \times 100$$

$$\text{Item difficulty} = .64$$

This means that 64% of the individuals in this analysis answered the item correctly. Therefore, this test item can be judged as being moderately difficult. The closer the item difficulty is to 0, the more difficult the item.

To compute the item discrimination, use the following procedure.

$$\text{Item discrimination} = \frac{R_u - R_l}{\frac{1}{2} T}$$

R_u = number of students with correct answer in the upper group.
R_l = number of students with correct answer in the lower group.
T = total.

The analysis for this would require subtracting the number of persons who completed the item correctly in the lower group from the number of persons in the upper group who answered the item correctly and then dividing by one half of the total number of persons included in the analysis.

$$\text{Item discrimination} = \frac{12 - 6}{\frac{1}{2} (28)}$$

$$\text{Item discrimination} = .43$$

This indicates a moderate degree of discrimination. If all the students in the upper group answered the item correctly and all the students in the lower group answered the item incorrectly that would show a perfect discrimination of 1.

Item difficulty and discrimination power are commonly employed statistics used by educators. Howard (1985) offers the Rasch

Model as an alternative to classical test theory. To date, this model has not been generally applied by the nursing education population. It is offered as an alternative, however. Those interested in using the Rasch Model are directed to Howard's article.

Quality of Distracters

The last activity that the test developer should complete on all items is a review of the distracters; this will assist in determining the success of the overall question. According to Gronlund (1981), the evaluation of the effectiveness of distracters in each item is a measure of the attractiveness of each of the incorrect alternatives. If too many students in the upper group picked a particular distracter, then one can cautiously deduce that the distracter was misleading. In completing item analyses, it is essential for the teacher to be aware that with another sample the item analysis may change. The test developer may wish to keep particular items in the test despite the apparent failure to measure specific content. An example of when this may occur is in a situation in which a question is written to test material in readings not addressed in class. In this case, the faculty member may opt to leave the item in the test even though a significant number of students in the upper group missed the item.

Most colleges and universities have statistical packages available that will compute the operations suggested earlier. Student ranking, numerical grade, item discrimination, item difficulty, and information on each response usually are readily available to the nurse educator who desires them.

Other types of objective tests include short answer or completion, alternative response, and matching. These types of examinations are particularly suited for testing the lower levels of Bloom's cognitive domains. Most measurement texts offer guidelines for constructing each of these types of exams.

Other Evaluation Strategies

In addition to objective testing, the nurse educator has the opportunity to use other types of theoretical evaluation strategies. These include having the student take essay examinations, write papers, develop class projects, and execute group or individual presentations. Any one of these strategies will help students who do not take objective tests well to demonstrate their level of competence in a specific content area. Additionally, these methods of evaluation offer students the opportunity to demonstrate their skills relative to the higher levels of Bloom's taxonomy. When developing an examination that will evaluate all levels of Bloom's taxonomy a combination of multiple choice, essay, and short answers will be required.

Two of the concerns raised about the use of the methods described earlier is that they are time-consuming to correct and have the potential to be subjective measures of student outcomes. Both of these issues warrant consideration; however, one must question the purpose of evaluation in deciding which evaluation method to use. For instance, if the purpose of an evaluation measure is to determine if a student can compare and contrast two types of nursing care delivery systems, this outcome is best measured in a way other than an objective multiple-choice examination. Even though the grading of an essay question necessitates additional faculty time, it would give the students the opportunity to compare and contrast and, therefore, be more appropriate to this learning objective.

If faculty members offer concerns about the subjective nature of grading another type of evaluation method, mechanisms can be developed to limit this problem. For instance, if one is using a paper to evaluate students' abilities to analyze material, criteria can be written for the paper, and a second reader can be employed. Nichols and Miller (1984) report a study in which they measured interrater reliability for grading of comprehensive examinations. Their findings and conclusions could be used to develop similar formats for presentations, essay exams, and student projects. Faculty should not shy away from the use of methods other than multiple choice objective testing, but should approach them with an open mind and an attitude of support for the student. Evaluation should not be used to find students errors but rather to acknowledge their level of achievement and direct future study.

Normative Versus Criterion-Referenced Evaluation

One issue concerning evaluation measures that faculty frequently face is whether or not the evaluation should be normative or criterion referenced in nature. Normative evaluation implies that the grades of the group tested are distributed in a normative or bell-shaped curve. Students' scores or grades are based on the abilities of the overall group. For example, 10 students complete a presentation and their grades are 98, 97, 95, 91, 87, 84, 80, 76, 70, and 68. The mean for this group is 84.3. The standard deviation is 10. Because most of the test scores will fall within 2 standard deviations of the mean, the grades might cluster as follows: 98 (A), 97 (B), 95 (B), 91 (C), 87 (C), 84 (C), 80 (C), 76 (D), 70 (D), and 68 (F). As can be seen from this example in a normative grading schema, most test scores would cluster around the center, or C, and grades would follow the normal bell-curve pattern.

Criterion-referenced evaluation, conversely, establishes a criterion that must be reached to meet a standard. Using the preceding example, if the criterion for an A were 92 to 100; for a B, 85 to 91; for a C, 78 to 84; for a D, 70 to 77; and for a F, less than 70, the grades would cluster differently. In this case there would be three A's, two B's, three C's, one D, and one F.

Depending on whether normative or criterion-referenced evaluation is chosen, the outcome could be very different. Theoretically, when using normative evaluation criteria, an entire class could fail an assignment with scores of 70 or less and still receive a passing grade.

Advantages and disadvantages arise with each approach to evaluation. It is important that the nurse educator know the advantages and disadvantages of each approach as well as the principles on which it is based because the choice of which evaluation approach to use rests with the educators who implement it.

Clinical Evaluation Measures

Much has been written about what Wooley (1977) has described as "the long and tortured history of clinical evaluation" (p. 308). It appears, however, that nurse educators continue to deliberate the merits and pitfalls of a variety of ways to evaluate students in the clinical area. The current nursing literature abounds with discussions and research reports related to clinical evaluation. Many of these reports suggest that nurse educators remain uncomfortable with the clinical evaluation aspect of their role. Indeed, the fact that so much has been written about clinical evaluation leads one to suspect that clinical evaluation makes nurse educators uncomfortable because of the lack of control and the subjectiveness of the measure.

Heard frequently are nurse educators' discussions of potential legal liability related to their role in the clinical area, which also causes a degree of uneasiness about the clinical experience itself. Related to this are comments reflecting potential legal action by students based on subjective evaluations. Fowler and Heater (1983) report cases in which the courts have upheld faculty rights to decide what constitutes professional practice without endless lists of behavioral objectives. Still, faculty members often remain uncomfortable.

Numerous articles are available detailing development of clinical evaluation tools that reduce subjectivity and assist the faculty members in making clearer determinations of student progress (Cottrell, et al., 1986; Higgins & Ochsner, 1989; Hillegas & Valentine, 1986; Jackson, Mead, & Moore, 1984; Novak, 1988; Pavlish, 1987; Stecchi, Woltman, Wall-Haas, Heggestad, & Zier, 1983; Tower & Majewski, 1987). Still, questions arise, and new tools continue to be developed. It is important for the nurse educator to accept and become comfortable with the subjective nature of clinical evaluation. If evaluation is viewed as an important learning tool by both faculty and students, some of the anxiety related to carrying it out might be reduced.

Recently, nurse educators have called for a curriculum revolution (Bevis, 1988; Chinn, 1988; Corcoran & Tanner, 1988; Diekelmann, 1988; Moccia, 1988; Munhall, 1988; Tanner, 1988; Watson, 1988). This revolution calls for an assessment of the way students are educated for the practice of nursing. In fact, if the way students are educated undergoes revolutionary changes, so must evaluation practices, particularly those related to clinical evaluation. As assessment and evaluation are carried out, nurse educators need to become comfortable in their respective roles and develop strategies that support their evaluative role.

One of the ways to begin to exercise the role of evaluator is to understand what it is that is expected of a beginning practitioner. This knowledge can be gleaned by reading the literature but also by watching practicing nurses and listening to nursing administration colleagues who work with neophyte nurses on a regular basis. Defining a goal and helping the student move toward that goal is one very valuable way to feel successful as a teacher and evaluator. Part of the nurse educator role in the clinical area is the role of teacher, a fact that should not be lost during the day-to-day functioning in patient care areas.

It is important that educators not focus solely on the evaluation role nor execute the evaluation process relying solely on behavioral objectives. As Malek (1988) states, "faculty must be aware of the limitation placed on evaluation when prestated objectives are the primary source of performance criteria. Comprehensive evaluation occurs best when natural interactions are guided and not bound by behavioral objectives" (p. 36). Clinical teaching faculty must free themselves from old patterns and move in the direction of facilitating student progress rather than concentrating on evaluating every behavior.

It is the contention of the authors that students will rise to the expectations set for them. If students are treated in positive, supportive ways, they will become the type of practitioners of whom nurse educators can be proud. If they are treated in demeaning and punitive ways, students will find ways to avoid interactions with faculty. Eluding faculty will limit learning opportunities that ultimately will result in loss of valuable experiences. Providing positive comments to learners will promote their confidence and will have the added benefit of making the clinical learning and evaluation process pleasant.

Contracting

One of the ways to facilitate evaluation of students is to make them part of the process. Assisting students in the development of strategies to direct their own learning experience enhances goal attainment. Most adults prefer to have some degree of control over activities in which they participate. Self-evaluation is offered as one of the strategies to facilitate feelings of empowerment in the evaluation situation. Recommended as a specific way to enhance students' feelings of control is the use of contracts.

Contracts are useful in the development of learning strategies and evaluation measurement in both the classroom and clinical areas. Beare (1985) and Sasmor (1984) offer ways to develop clinical grading contracts. Generally, this strategy provides students with the opportunity to develop their own learning objectives based on the objectives of the course. It also provides them with the freedom to construct their own evaluation measures. Use of contracting as a teaching and evaluation strategy assists students in developing practices that will be useful in the classroom and in the workplace. Educators may wish to consider contracting as an alternative to the typically used pedagogical model that places the teacher as the ultimate knower and views students as empty vessels awaiting occupation.

SUMMARY

This discussion has explored the evaluation process, suggesting ways of constructing objective and subjective evaluation strategies, and described statistical operations as they related to objective test construction. In addition, strategies for becoming an effective clinical evaluator have been offered.

There are a variety of ways to measure different types of learning outcomes, and it is important for nurse educators to remember that the final choices for which methods to employ rests with them. Although evaluation is frequently viewed in a negative context, it is suggested that if educators view it as a growth experience for the student and themselves, the process will be far less threatening to both students and educators.

REFERENCES

American Psychological Association, Inc. (1985). *Standards for educational and psychological testing.* Washington, DC: Author.

Anastasi, A. (1982). *Psychological testing* (5th ed.). New York; Macmillan.

Beare, P. (1985). The clinical contract—An approach to competency based clinical learning and evaluation. *Journal of Nursing Education,* 24(2), 75–77.

Bevis, E. O. (1988). New directions for a new age. In *Curriculum revolution: Mandate for change* (pp. 27–52). New York: National League for Nursing.

Bloom, B. S. (Ed.). (1956). *Taxonomy of educational objectives : Handbook I: Cognitive domain.* New York: Longman.

Chinn, P. (1988, December). *Feminist pedagogy in nursing education.* Paper presented at the Fifth National Conference on Nursing Education, Chicago, IL.

Corcoran, S. A., & Tanner, C. (1988). Implications of clinical judgement research for teaching. In *Curriculum revolution: Mandate for change* (pp. 159–176). New York: National League for Nursing.

Cottrell, B. H., Cox, B. H., Kelsey, S. J., Ritchie, P. J., Rumph, E. A., & Shannahan, M. K. (1986). A clinical evaluation tool for nursing students using nursing process. *Journal of Nursing Education*, 25(7), 270–274.

Diekelmann, N. (1988). Curriculum revolution: A theoretical and philosophical mandate for change. In *Curriculum revolution: Mandate for change* (pp. 137–158). New York: National League for Nursing.

Flynn, M. K., & Reese, J. L. (1988). Development and evaluation of classroom tests: A practical application. *Journal of Nursing Education*, 27(2), 61–65.

Fowler, G. A., & Heater, B. (1983). Guidelines for clinical evaluation. *Journal of Nursing Education*, 22(9), 402–404.

Frisbie, D. A. (1983). Testing achievement beyond the knowledge level. *Journal of Nursing Education*, 22(6), 228–231.

Gronlund, N. E. (1981). *Measurement and evaluation in teaching* (4th ed). New York: Macmillan.

Higgins, B., & Ochsner, S. (1989). Two approaches to clinical evaluation. *Nurse Educator*, 14(2), 8–11.

Hillegas, K. B., & Valentine, S. (1986). Development and evaluation of a summative clinical grading tool. *Journal of Nursing Education*, 25(5), 218–220.

Howard, E. P. (1985). Applying the Rasch model to test administration. *Journal of Nursing Education*, 24(8), 340–343.

Huben–Stanton, M. P. (1983). Objective test construction: A must for nursing educators. *Journal of Nursing Education*, 22(8), 338–339.

Jackson, S. S., Mead, J. E., & Moore, J. B. (1984). Evaluating clinical fitness. *Journal of Nursing Education*, 23(8), 364–366.

Krathwohl, D. R., Bloom, B. S., & Masia, B. B. (1964). *Taxonomy of educational objectives: Book 2: Affective domain*. New York: Longman.

Litwack, L., Linc, L., & Bower, D. (1985). *Evaluation in nursing: Principles and practice*. New York: National League for Nursing.

Malek, C. J. (1988). Clinical evaluation: Challenging tradition. *Nurse Educator*, 13(6), 34–37.

Moccia, P. (1988, December).*Curriculum reconceptualization: Integrating the voices of revolution*. Paper presented at the Fifth National Conference on Nursing Education, Chicago, IL.

Munhall, P. (1988). Curriculum revolution: A social mandate for change. In *Curriculum revolution: Mandate for change* (pp. 217–230). New York: National League for Nursing.

Nichols, E. G., & Miller, G. K. (1984). Interreader agreement on comprehensive essay examinations. *Journal of Nursing Education*, 23(2), 64–69.

Novak, S. (1988). An effective clinical evaluation tool. *Journal of Nursing Education, 27*(2), 83–84.

Pavlish, C. (1987). A model for clinical performance evaluation. *Journal of Nursing Education, 26*(8), 338–339.

Sasmor, J. L. (1984). Contracting for clinical. *Journal of Nursing Education, 23*(4), 171–173.

Stecchi, J. M., Woltman, S. J., Wall–Hass, C., Heggestad, B., & Zier, M. (1983). Comprehensive approach to clinical evaluation: One teaching team's solution to clinical evaluation of students in multiple settings. *Journal of Nursing Education, 22*(1), 38–46.

Tanner, C. (1988). Curriculum revolution: The practice mandate. In *Curriculum revolution: Mandate for change* (pp. 201–216). New York: National League for Nursing.

Tower, B. L., & Majewski, T. V. (1987). Behaviorally based clinical evaluation. *Journal of Nursing Education, 26*(3), 120–123.

Watson, J. (1988). A case study: Curriculum in transition. In *Curriculum revolution: Mandate for change* (pp. 1–8). New York: National League for Nursing.

Wooley, A. S. (1977). The long and tortured history of clinical evaluation. *Nursing Outlook, 25*(5), 308–315.

UNIT IV
Student-Related
Issues for
Faculty Members

LETTERS

Dear Terry,

A whole new issue has developed for me in recent weeks; one I'm not sure I have ever thought about specifically in the past. I know I was of the opinion that once I became a nursing educator everything would just fall into place. Well, it *is* falling, but certainly not as I had envisioned it!

This week during a clinical experience, I became acutely aware of the multiplicity of responsibilities I have. As an educator, I am not only responsible for the actions of the students I teach, but I also have a responsibility to the profession of nursing, the school where I teach, the department of nursing within the university, the clients for whom the students care, the agency where we have clinical experience, and the parents who are spending tremendous amounts of money for their sons' and daughters' education, which I'm responsible for providing. When outlined in this way, I feel this tremendous burden. But before I get too carried away, let me start by telling you a little about my present situation.

One of my students, Susan, is doing very poorly. She is in serious academic difficulty, and she has a great deal of work to do to pass the course.

In class, Susan takes notes feverishly, struggling to get every word; she is quite attentive. Despite this, however, she has failed every exam except for one. In the clinical area, she also appears to put forth her absolute best effort, but, again, she is functioning at a level that is much lower than her peers, and that is not at the level expected by the objectives. I must admit I can't believe she has made it to this point in the nursing program! I suspect that a number of factors have influenced her continuing even though her academic and clinical performances are substandard: enrollments are lower in the university in general and in our department specifically, and there is pressure to keep students in the system; faculty members seem to have an attitude that beginning students can't fail; the fear of legal action is rampant. (By the way, Susan is a minority student.)

I suppose the issue for me is the multitude of factors that conflict with one another. First and foremost, I have a commitment to the profession. I believe that nursing needs standards, and in order to uphold those standards, we need accountable, responsible, intelligent clinicians. (I'm sure my adjectives could go on and on, but you know what I mean, don't you?)

This commitment to quality nursing, however, seems to be at odds with an earnest desire to support and nurture individuals who choose to enter the profession. For example, I want to allow Susan the time she needs to learn, but at what point do I say, "It's time for an evaluation of just what you can and can't do, and what you do and don't know"? What about prior learning? Do I need to reevaluate it? There seems to be some very important knowledge that Susan has either forgotten or that she never learned. Underlying all of these questions is a basic need on my part not to be an ogre. I do not want to teach by the evaluation method. Help!

There are other issues. Susan is really a very lovely young woman. Her family has been in this country only for about five years, and all three of her family members hold a variety of odd jobs to keep Susan in school. Obviously, she and they have come a very long way in a short period. How can I destroy their dreams by giving her a failing grade?

Susan tells me she studies all the time, and I believe her. I have counseled her almost weekly, and I recommended a tutor as soon as her problem was identified; however, I'm afraid it will not be enough. The tutoring center reports that she comes to all of her assigned appointments with her work done, and that during the sessions, she works extremely hard. But she still has not improved her test scores or level of clinical performance.

When I spoke to one of my colleagues about this situation, she said it wasn't worth the hassle it would cause if I failed her in the course. She told me just to let Susan go on in the program. Another colleague suggested that a discrimination suit might result because of her minority status and the fact that I recommended tutoring so early in the semester.

I'm so confused. Do I follow my peers' advice, or do I carry out my responsibilities as my "gut" dictates and take the chance of suffering the consequences?

Other issues that seem to be in conflict with one another are the client's right to safe, efficient, and effective care and the student's need to learn in a conducive, nonthreatening environment. How can both of these goals be met simultaneously? How can I create a nonthreatening environment, given the recent changes in the health care scene? How long can a client who is being cared for by a student be expected to "tolerate" the neophyte's actions?

I raise these questions because Susan is very awkward and disorganized at the bedside. Added to that is the fact that her English pronunciation is poor and her accent obvious. Clients sometimes verbalize their annoyance at her lack of skill in carrying out even the most basic skills.

I have sent Susan back to the learning laboratory to practice the skills that she cannot perform competently. Great! Then what happens? She returns to the clinical unit with a slip of paper indicating successful completion of the required learning objective, but on demonstration of the skill in the hospital, she is unsuccessful two out of three times! On that infrequent occasion when she *is* successful, she looks up at me and smiles widely with genuine enthusiasm for her triumph. I want to cry when I congratulate her on her achievement, but at the same time need to inform her that one correct demonstration out of three is not an acceptable standard in the program or in the profession. She then begins to cry and verbalize her hostility toward me. Surprisingly, she is very eloquent in her statements about my lack of caring. Susan believes that I "pick on her."

One other part of this problem is related to the other students in the clinical setting. Some verbalize their impatience with me for the time I spend with Susan, and others just demonstrate all sorts of hostile behavior toward Susan. In essence, they are very angry about the limited instruction and support *they* are getting because of the time I feel compelled to spend with Susan. They have every right to be angry! Yet I do not believe Susan is safe, nor can she be left alone.

It's times like this one when I wonder whether I really want to teach as much as I think I do. This feels like a "no-win" situation. I see myself as a very committed nurse educator. But to be honest with you—and with my-self—I am *very* confused about what I want and what I believe. Please write soon and give me some of your wonderful insight!

Dear Helen,

It was, as usual, so very nice to hear from you. I'm only sorry the student you wrote about is causing you such worry.

Isn't it amazing that the people we are in this thing called education for—the students—can be precisely the people who make us think, "What am I doing here?!" As I think back on the literally hundreds of students I have known over the years, who is it that comes to mind?

In some ways it's the students who failed a course or who couldn't progress to the next level because they didn't have Microbiology, or the students who made such a fuss about their clinical placements, or the ones with whom I felt a personality conflict. But the students who *really* stick out in my mind, though, are the ones who grew so much over the semester, or the ones who really got "turned on" to nursing after their senior practicum experience.

It seems to me these positive experiences surely outweigh the negative ones. The negative ones—like the situation you described—are so draining, though! They do begin to make you question your competence, your judgment, your sense of fairness, and even your own worth. But, Helen, if you yield to all the pressures you're feeling, you'll question those things even more. You'll question your own integrity as well.

Yes, when students fail, they're angry. If you think about it, it's almost as if they go through the grieving process; they get very angry, they suffer a sense of loss (of self-esteem, of immediate goals, etc.), they want to bargain to change the grade so they pass, and so on. No doubt, it's a *very* difficult situation for them. If you follow this theme of the grieving process through to its conclusion, though, one hopes that the students move to acceptance; all the threats are just idle ones.

Over the years, I have had to give students some very bad news, namely, that they did not pass a paper or a course, or that they couldn't progress to the next level in the program. Invariably, their initial response was anger, but do you know what? Many of those students made a special effort to come back to me later and thank me. Yes, thank me! They've come back and said, "You know, I was devastated when I saw that failure, but when I re-read the paper and your comments on it, looked again at the evaluation criteria, and allowed myself to be honest, I realized you were absolutely right and justified. I'm here to thank you—funny as that sounds—and to ask you where I can go for help." For students who failed a course, comments like the following have not been uncommon: "The thought of having to repeat the course and be 'out of synch' with my friends was devastating, but I decided to repeat it anyway, and I've found out a few things about myself. I found out I really *didn't* know the material, I *hadn't* put as much effort into the course as I should have, and my friends are *still* my friends, even though we're not in the same classes. I've also found I grew up a lot as a result of this experience, and maybe I'll be even a better, more mature nurse."

Now, those may sound like very mature responses, but they are real! They have come from undergraduate students. You know, sometimes I think we grossly underestimate our students.

You may be thinking this is all well and good, but what do I do about Susan. In a nutshell, I'd say, "Stick to your guns" and continue to uphold high standards of performance. You also have to do some soul searching to make sure you aren't being biased.

You are under a lot of pressure, Helen . . . pressure from Susan, your peers, the patients, the agency staff, Susan's parents, yourself . . . and my guess is you feel all alone. For what it's worth, I support you, and my guess is that many of your faculty colleagues do, too, although they may not be willing to express such support.

You mentioned your surprise that Susan had gotten as far as she did. Well, maybe she shouldn't have passed sophomore year, but you can't change that now, so don't make yourself crazy over it. You can, however, get your faculty group to look at expected standards of performance at each level, what is meant by an A, B, or C, or perhaps institute a comprehensive exam at the end of each level. Those are the kinds of questions that need to be asked now.

Let's get back to Susan. It sounds to me as if you've been objective in your assessments of her: you've noted her attentiveness in class, her willingness to give it her all, her joy at doing something correctly, and her apparent love of nursing. You've been clear about her weaknesses and problems and have sent her back to the lab as necessary, sent her for tutoring, and spent a good deal of time with her. Finally, you've been honest with her about the problems with her clinical performance. I don't know what else you can do.

Your other clinical students are quite justified in feeling neglected; given all the time Susan has needed, these students probably have *not* received the attention they deserve. It's not fair that they are left to "fend for themselves" because of Susan. If Susan is not prepared for her clinical assignment (something you assess at the very start of the clinical day, obviously), then she should not be allowed to be involved with patient care. If she can't be involved in patient care, then she can't meet the clinical objectives.

You need to be sure you aren't assigning Susan to care for patients who require knowledge and skills beyond that needed by other students' patients, that you aren't asking her questions that are different from those you ask other students, and that you aren't expecting her to perform like a senior student or a graduate nurse. Once you're convinced you are treating Susan in the same way you treat other students (and maybe it would help if you talked this over with someone), then you need to document carefully and objectively Susan's (and all other students'!) clinical performance abilities and keep Susan informed of her progress. If she fails, remember it's *she* who has failed to meet the objectives, not *you* who has failed her.

In your letter, you said one of your colleagues said it wasn't worth the hassle to give Susan a failing grade. I disagree totally! (And from your letter, it sounds like you disagree, too.) It *is* worth the hassle. It's worth it to Susan, because if she is allowed to continue, she will be placed in increasingly complex situations and be expected to make more decisions independently; if she doesn't have the foundation or ability to function in that way, she'll be frustrated. Of course, it's worth it to the patients, who have the right to be cared for by competent nurses. It's worth it to the profession, particularly because today's crises require competent, articulate, and truly professional nurses in practice; it will not serve any of us well to have a cadre of practitioners who cannot think or provide top-notch patient care. It's also worth it, I would think, to your school because its reputation will not be well served when the nursing community sees that students are passed even when they aren't able to perform as expected, simply because it's the easiest way out.

Most important, however, Helen, is that it's worth it to you. You are the one who is going to have to live with what you do. If you pass Susan knowing she really deserved to fail, will you feel good about yourself? Will you be able to face your colleagues and other students? Will you ever have confidence in your judgment as a clinical teacher again? My guess is the answer to these questions is "no."

I'm not saying that faculty should do things simply because they think it's best for them. Far from it! Indeed, I think too much of that goes on already! What I *am* saying is that faculty members should do what they believe—in their expert judgment as educators—is the right and most responsible way to act.

It is not an easy job being a nurse educator. I think you knew that when you took your position. You *do* have a tremendous amount of responsibility and a great many "audiences" to whom you have to play. When it's in you blood, though, there still is nothing else you'd rather do. I think any job in nursing is a difficult, demanding, highly responsible one—just the details are different from one job to the next. When you are dealing with people—and that's what we do all the time—you can't control them, you can't program them, and you can't predict their every behavior. But isn't that precisely why we went into nursing in the first place? . . . and into teaching?

You've been very successful as a clinician, well prepared to be a teacher, and functioned beautifully as an educator; you're also asking the right kinds of questions about the situations you're in. Don't doubt your judgments so much. You know you have to make many difficult decisions, and Susan's situation is one of them. I know you'll do the best thing, even if it's not the easy way out.

Well, enough rambling. Remember what I said at the start of this letter. The students who do not do well are cause for concern and do make us question why we're in teaching; however, there are many students who will do very well, grow before your very eyes, and eventually make significant contributions to nursing and patient care. Don't let all those rewarding experiences be overshadowed.

Take care and keep in touch.

10

Traditional and Diverse Learners in Nursing: Admission, Progression, and Maintenance of Standards

The nursing profession has been faced with several external changes that have transformed the ability of nurse educators to attract qualified applicants to the field. Green (1987) highlighted the results of the Cooperative Institutional Research Program (CIRP), which surveyed college freshmen to determine a profile of American education. Specifically the survey identifies the traits, characteristics, aspirations, values, and expectations of individuals entering postsecondary educational institutions. The results of the survey provide important information about what the nursing education community can expect from students entering nursing programs.

The CIRP findings indicated that college age students of the 1980s were more materialistic and less interested in altruistic careers. They wanted high-status professions that would yield significant dollar incomes, and the majors they preferred were business, law, medicine, science, and engineering. Freshman women's attitudes toward careers were more supportive of job equality than they were 20 years ago. In addition, "women . . . outnumber[ed] men in the undergraduate population" (Green, 1987, p. 249). There is no evidence to suggest that students of the 1990s or of the early part of the next century will be very different from those of the 1980s.

What does all this mean for nursing education? Today, although the late 1980s and early 1990s have shown a slight increase in applications to nursing programs when compared to the early 1980s, there are still fewer high school students choosing nursing as a career than was the case 20 or more years ago. Green (1987) reported "in 1986–1987, the number of freshmen women in four-year colleges and universities planning to pursue medical careers [was] larger than the number of women interested in nursing careers by more than 5000 students" (p. 250). Needless to say, this places ongoing demands on the nursing education system to recruit and retain qualified candidates. In addition, according to the College Board (Farrell, 1988), the average combined Scholastic Aptitude Test (SAT) score for students intending to pursue nursing as a career choice was 689 in 1985. This represented a 217-point decline from the national average SAT for that year. How has nursing education dealt with shifting enrollments and less academically prepared students and remained a viable profession?

A report of an NLN study noted "shrinking applicant pools are forcing programs to lower admissions standards and to offer large doses of remediation to the students they accept" (Rosenfeld, 1987, p. 283). Is this the way nursing will cope with the shifting demographics of individuals pursuing nursing as a career?

Nursing has several ways to deal with the challenges that face the nursing educational system. Many institutions maintained standards despite lowered enrollments during the 1980s and accepted a smaller student body. Other schools have lowered admission standards. Many other nursing education programs have been forced to lower admission standards, but have developed remedial programs to maximize student potentials. Still other institutions have bypassed this issue altogether by seeking nontraditional markets for potential students. All of these strategies are directed at maintaining the number of students in programs of nursing, and their impact is only now being felt in nursing programs throughout this country.

ADMISSION OF TRADITIONAL NURSING STUDENTS

The change in demographics has created the need for change in recruitment strategies. Concomitant with any change in recruitment plans is the need to address what adjustments will be needed to meet the demands of educating students with backgrounds different from those which have been traditionally encountered in nursing education programs. Nursing is now dealing with a potential market of students who are "shopping" for educational opportunities that will meet their needs. Students increasingly verbalize an awareness of their needs and rights as they relate to the educational experience. Nursing faculty members need to be similarly aware of the needs and rights of the students being admitted to their programs.

Since the 1960s, students in higher education have been more vocal about their rights as they relate to the student experience. Because of the demand for students' rights, most colleges and universities have sought legal consultation and developed specific policies that address criteria for student admission, promotion, and graduation. These data are published in school catalogs to serve as an easy reference. In view of what is perceived as a need for additional requirements, some schools and departments within colleges and universities develop specific admission, promotion, and graduation criteria for students in their respective programs. On many college campuses, nursing is one of the programs that frequently includes additional criteria.

Typically, basic admission criteria for nursing program admission are similar to that for the college or university including documentation of completion of secondary schooling with a grade point average (GPA) of 2.0 or better, acceptable performance on either American College Test (ACT) or SAT tests, and evidence of ability to complete the program of study. In addition, specific admission criteria for particular nursing programs might include a writing sample, above-average grades in high school science and math courses, GPA of 2.5 or better, and an interview. Some nursing faculty groups have identified these requirements as necessary screening mechanisms to assure the acceptance of well-qualified student nursing candidates.

Admission committees at the university-college level or nursing department review the materials submitted, and typically recommend or deny admission to the prospective candidates. Given the current decrease in the applicant pool, many colleges and universities as well as the nursing departments within them have had to rethink their admission policies. Lowering admission criteria, however, may not be the most appropriate action to take. Several studies (Glick, McClelland, & Yang, 1986; Payne & Duffy, 1986; Quick, Krupa, & Whitley,

1985; Whitley & Chadwick, 1986; Yocum & Scherubel, 1985) have documented the predictiveness of "pre-admission variables such as high school performance [both GPA and class rank], the verbal and mathematics components of the [SAT], or the multiple components of the [ACT]" (Jenks, Selekman, Bross, & Paquet, 1989, p. 113), and student success and performance on the NCLEX-RN. Based on this research, it is shortsighted to reduce standards without further study of preadmission variables.

Some schools that have maintained standards have faced faculty retrenchment. Colleges and universities are businesses that derive a significant proportion of their operating budgets from tuitions. If student populations are not available in sufficient numbers to support the faculty, then faculty positions need to be eliminated.

Lost faculty lines may not bode well for nursing education on campuses, but the larger question facing nursing education administrators before the loss of these positions is to what end the nursing education division will go to maintain faculty positions and provide a continuing student pool. Lay and professional literature documents the increasing demand and lagging supply of qualified practitioners to assume nursing positions. Now more than ever before, nursing education is faced with the challenge of recruiting and sustaining a number of nontraditional learners including second-career students, registered nurse students, and mature adults seeking their first academic degree. All of these groups come with their own unique needs and all require special attention.

ADMISSION OF NONTRADITIONAL STUDENTS

Nursing shortages have occurred sporadically throughout the history of American nursing. During the 1980s, nursing faced one of the low points in its ability to recruit qualified individuals. Recently, nursing has seen a shift in enrollments. The NLN ("Trends Are," 1990) reported an 8.9% increase in enrollments during the fall of 1989. Although this report demonstrates an improvement, there are several reasons why the problem exists. Reduced numbers of 18-year-olds available for college, more job opportunities for women, and a poor image of the nursing profession are just a few. In view of these factors limiting the availability of prospective students as well as the increased demands for nursing personnel created by technological advances, nurse educators have been forced to seek nursing student applicants from typically untapped sources.

First-time adult college students and second-career students now represent a larger proportion of the prospective nursing student pool than has been typical in the past. It is shortsighted for nursing programs to use high school records as part of the admission process for this group of students. High school records of adults over 21 years of age give little information about current abilities. For these students it is useful to use other measures such as an experience and educational portfolio that may provide a more appropriate way to assess their potential for success in a nursing program. Interviews also are valuable in giving prospective nontraditional students the opportunity to share their life experiences, strengths, and potentials.

Encouraging first-time adult college students to take some courses outside of the nursing major before applying for matriculation is another way of gauging their ability. If students have the opportunity to move slowly back into formalized education, they will have the added benefit of gaining their self-confidence in the academic environment before moving directly into their chosen field.

Another group of nontraditional individuals seeking admission to nursing programs are individuals with a completed degree in another area. Again it would be inappropriate to use second-degree students' high school records. Depending on how recently the first degree was obtained, success in the first major can be used to determine whether or not the prospective student has the potential to complete the nursing degree. Similar to the first-time adult college student, it would be most useful to have second-degree students develop education and experience portfolios to evaluate their ability to complete the program.

Another related challenge arises in assessment of foreign students' records for admission to the nursing program. Evaluation of these students' transcripts is more complex because the secondary schooling completed in foreign countries may not be comparable by the standards used for American students. The admissions office or office of international studies can offer assistance to the nursing department in evaluating foreign students' records. Criteria for determining admission may have to be flexible to provide students with the opportunity to enter the nursing program.

Minority students from the United States are another group of students that present admission committees with a challenge. Allen, Nunley, and Scott-Warner (1988) conducted research on the recruitment and retention of black students and found that issues of recruitment and retention for minority students, and in particular black students, is different from those that typically affect the recruitment and retention of white students. This group of investigators found that the barriers to admission included poor secondary preparation, limited recruitment of black students, inadequate financial aid, lack of encouragement by high school counselors to attend college, perceived hostile attitudes towards blacks in colleges, and a feeling of being unwelcome on university campuses.

In addition, Boyle (1986) found different predictors of success for minority nursing student populations than are usually found in nonminority populations. In this study, performance on the state board examination was used as the outcome variable. Entering GPA, ACT, high school rank (HSRANK), number of college credit hours prior to program admission (HRSPTA), high school GPA, age at admission, index of applicant motivation, and related experience, were investigated as predictors of success in the state board examination. Boyle found that ACT scores were the strongest predictor of success on the state board examination for all minorities, followed by HSRANK and HRSPTA, offering "some explanatory power, particularly for black students" (p. 191).

These studies suggest that it is valuable for college and nursing department admission committees to look closely at a variety of indicators when making admission decisions. ACT or SAT scores provide admissions committees with one indication of potential success for the rigors of nursing programs. Minimum admission level scores may be established, but such decisions should be made based on the current research related to the particular individual about whom a decision is being made. Additionally, admission committees should develop a variety of requirements based on the needs of the individual being reviewed. For example, a GPA of 2.3 from high school completed 25 years ago, science and math grades less than 2.5 from the same period, and no SAT or ACT scores would probably disqualify a

45-year-old learner from admission to most nursing programs if standard admission criteria were applied. Provisional admission, however, may provide the adult learner with the opportunity to demonstrate current abilities.

Another group of learners for whom admission criteria may need to be modified are returning registered nurse students. These individuals come with unique learning needs and must be supported in movement toward their personal career goals. In addition to review of standard admission information, admission committees should include data relative to the RN student's current employment roles, progress toward career goals, life experience, and evidence of ongoing education, such as conference attendance and references. Furthermore, schools of nursing have the ability to use standardized tests based on the background of RN students to evaluate their academic abilities (Dixon, 1989).

The most important point to be made related to the recruitment and selection of students for a nursing program is that college and nursing department admission committees must carefully review the records of prospective applicants and ensure that a variety of sources of information are used in making admission decisions. Although it would be disastrous for all nursing programs to significantly lower their admissions standards across the board, it will be equally disastrous to eliminate potential candidates who do not seem to meet the standards because of nontraditional entry points. Nursing educators must maintain standards for the profession. It will be necessary for nurse educators to become flexible and creative in their approach to admitting individuals interested in nursing as a career.

TRADITIONAL STUDENTS

The decline in the abilities of the freshman pool available for nursing education programs during the 1980s was documented earlier. Given these data, faculty need to ask: What mechanisms must be developed or implemented to maintain these students, in nursing programs and provide for their success as graduates?

Developing qualified practitioners of professional nursing is the commitment of nursing educators. In light of this commitment and awareness of differing levels of student abilities, it is vital to develop and enhance services that will ensure student success. Identification of what will be necessary to support students who are academically disadvantaged is the responsibility of all nursing faculty groups who choose to admit students of this type. If resources are unavailable within the college or university, then they must be made available through the nursing program. Students will require note-taking, study, and test-taking skills as well as paper-writing seminars. In addition, students may need reading and math remediation to complete the program requirements successfully. Nursing faculty must be cognizant of all the resources that are available and that may need to be made available to ensure student success in the program. In some schools, nursing faculty members have assumed responsibility for helping students develop note-taking, study, and test-taking skills, as well as math and reading remediation for their students as a way of maintaining programs. Because of the changing climate in which programs are operating today, this strategy has preserved faculty positions. There may be questions, however, that arise related to the expertise of nursing faculty for the provision of these services. Nursing faculty members have a responsibility to assume only those assignments for which they are prepared. If college or university administrations are requesting these services from nurse educators, then it is critical that faculty members have the opportunity to develop the needed skills.

Faculty members have a responsibility to help students toward realization of successful completion of the nursing program. Faculty members also have a responsibility to maintain the quality of care delivered to clients. With both of these obligations in mind, it is essential that nurse educators be aware of the variety of support services available within the college or university as well as which support services are expected from within the nursing department. Most public colleges and universities have a variety of support services available including counseling, assistance with study and test-taking skills, time-management workshops, and reading and writing laboratories. Cameron-Buccheri and Trygstad (1989) identify the services they believed essential in the retention of freshman students at the University of San Francisco. These services include freshmen orientation, one-to-one advisement during the first 6 weeks of the semester, identification of high-risk students during the first 2 weeks of school so early interventions can be made, planned opportunities for freshman students to meet, time-management and study-skills seminars during the first week of school, encouragement of group studying, and, if possible, enrollment in a nursing course during the first semester.

Lack of support services occurs most often in the small private colleges where resources may be limited. When services are not provided for students who need them, their academic success may be in jeopardy.

It is important that nursing faculty apprises students of expectations. Students should be provided with progression requirements on acceptance into the nursing program. At the beginning of a new course, students also should be informed about the requirements and grading policies of the course. Students who demonstrate difficulty in meeting the requirements of particular courses should be provided with faculty support and direction. If the problem is out of the area of expertise of the nursing faculty member, then the student should be referred to the appropriate skill center. Through early referral, chances for successful completion of coursework is improved.

Nursing educators also should be aware of and use the research on teaching-learning strategies. All students are not capable of being successful in a learning situation that requires learner passivity and evaluation based solely on teacher-made multiple-choice tests. Creativity in teaching and evaluation strategies can promote student learning. Faculty members should be supported within their academic unit in the development of a repertoire of creative teaching and evaluation methodologies. Through use of multiple teaching and evaluation strategies, nursing educators have the opportunity to meet the varied learning needs of diverse student groups and thereby enhance their chances of success in the program.

NONTRADITIONAL STUDENTS

To meet the needs of adult or nontraditional learners in nursing education programs, nursing faculty should first review the literature on the needs of these students. Faculty then should meet to discuss their perceptions of the learning needs of the nontraditional learner. Buckley (1980) found, for example, that the single most important factor in retention of black students is faculty commitment. This type of faculty commitment to teaching nontraditional learners has a significant impact on the success students are likely to enjoy.

Finally, opportunities should be made available to explore with the current or potential groups of adult learners what their perceived needs are. This can be done by using former and currently enrolled nontraditional students as an advisory group to the nursing education unit. It is likely that some of the needs identified include flexibility in scheduling, ways of meeting course requirements through nontraditional means such as learning portfolios, childcare, financial assistance, access to student services such as extended evening hours, and credit for past learning experiences. Obvious to some is that these are not requests made by the typical 18-year-old entering a nursing program. Given that most adult learners come with diverse backgrounds, there is a tremendous need to be sensitive to their life situations.

Many nontraditional students enroll in nursing programs with a hope of developing employable skills. While developing these skills, there is a need to continue to support themselves. Because there is limited financial assistance available for individuals seeking second careers on a part-time basis, maintenance of employment is a necessity for many.

In view of the need to support themselves, adult learners will be looking for flexibility in scheduling. Courses of study that offer credit for life experience and opportunities to challenge for credit are particularly sought by this group. In addition, traditional daytime clinical experiences may not meet the needs of this group. Opportunities to meet clinical requirements in a nontraditional manner, such as through evening or weekend experiences, may enhance retention of adult learners.

Many adult learners will be sensitive to what they perceive as differences between themselves and traditional students. In particular, they may identify that they do not think about education in the same way the traditional 18-year-old does. For the adult learner, education may not be viewed as a 4-year full-time commitment on the way to a first job. Also as a result of their absence from formal education, adult learners may feel insecure about reentry into the academic arena. Adult learners usually cannot meet a rigid academic schedule that does not support their need to work. With these reasons in mind, nursing educators interested in recruiting and retaining adult learners must develop strategies to enhance their learning experiences. They need support and guidance that considers their uniqueness as adult learners. Support groups and student services will need to be tailored to meet the needs of this population.

In addition to providing unique learning experiences for adult learners who are seeking their first professional degree, programs that offer second-degree students the opportunity to be granted credit for their past educational experience also are needed. Programs that specifically address the needs of second-degree students include Yale, Pace, University of Tennessee at Knoxville, McGill, Creighton, Case Western Reserve, Vanderbilt, and Emory. These institutions recognize the previous bachelor's degree and offer the master's degree as the first professional nursing degree. The perception of those who use this type of model for second-degree student learning is that it gives credit for the previous degree and provides an accelerated pathway into nursing.

Although all nursing programs may not be able to offer specific courses of study for all types of diverse learners, it is important to be aware that such programs exist. Advising nontraditional adult learners about programs that offer courses of study consistent with their personal learning objectives and needs is the responsibility of all educators.

The nursing profession is demonstrating a commitment to recruitment of adult learners as one means to increase the number of nursing students being educated. Nursing education faculty and administrators must retool to meet the needs of these students. Nurse educators must develop strategies that will facilitate the expeditious and successful completion of nursing program requirements by this group of students.

SUMMARY

The situation that nursing education faces related to changing enrollment patterns provides an opportunity for nursing professionals to re-examine recruitment and retention practices that are now in place. If nursing is interested in recruiting the most qualified candidates to move into professional practice positions, then it is imperative that strategies be developed that will most effectively meet the needs of a varied group of learners who choose programs with aspirations of becoming nurses. Nurse educators must look beyond the traditional 18-year-old market to enlist those adult learners who could contribute significantly to the profession.

Regarding maintenance of both traditional and nontraditional students in nursing programs, current programs of study must be reviewed to identify which admission and progression standards are essential and which are not realistic in today's marketplace. Nurse educators must strive to support students through the provision of services that will facilitate their successful completion of academic programs. Faculty must never lose sight of the fact that maintenance of quality nursing care begins with individuals prepared for the professional nursing role. Nurse educators must develop their personal nursing education expertise to cultivate the talents of those who would be nursing professionals.

Nursing is, indeed, in a time of great change. Nursing educators would be wise to seize the opportunities created by the current changes in supply and demand, and foster the successful development of programs that will guide the practice of nursing today and for the foreseeable future.

REFERENCES

Allen, M. E., Nunley, J. C., & Scott-Warner, M. (1988). Recruitment and retention of black students in baccalaureate nursing programs. *Journal of Nursing Education*, 27(3), 107–116.

Boyle, K. K. (1986). Predicting the success of minority students in baccalaureate nursing programs. *Journal of Nursing Education*, 25(5), 186–192.

Buckley, J. (1980). Faculty commitment to retention and recruitment of black students. *Nursing Outlook*, 28(2), 46–50.

Cameron-Buccheri, R., & Trygstad, L. (1989). Retaining freshman nursing students. *Nursing & Health Care*, 10(7), 389–393.

Dixon, A. Y. (1989). Project L.I.N.C.: An innovative model of educational mobility. *Nursing & Health Care*, 10(7), 399–402.

Farrell, J. (1988). The changing pool of candidates for nursing. *Journal of Professional Nursing*, 4(3), 145, 230.

Glick, O. J., McClelland, E., & Yang, C. (1986). NCLEX-RN: Predicting the performance of graduates of an integrated baccalaureate nursing program. *Journal of Professional Nursing, 2*(2), 98–103.

Green, K. C. (1987). The educational "pipeline" in nursing. *Journal of Professional Nursing, 3*(4), 247–257.

Jenks, J., Selekman, J., Bross, T., & Paquet, M. (1989). Success in NCLEX-RN: Identifying predictors and optimal time for intervention. *Journal of Nursing Education, 28*(3), 112–118.

Payne, M., & Duffy, M. (1986). An investigation of predictability of NCLEX scores of BSN graduates using academic predictors. *Journal of Professional Nursing, 2*(5), 326–332.

Quick, M., Krupa, K., & Whitley, T. (1985). Using admission data to predict success on the NCLEX-RN in a baccalaureate program. *Journal of Professional Nursing, 1*(6), 364–368.

Rosenfeld, P. (1987). Nursing education in crisis—A look at recruitment and retention. *Nursing & Health Care, 8*(5), 283–286.

Trends are encouraging, but the shortage isn't over yet. (1990). *Nursing & Health Care, 11*(6), 317.

Whitley, M., & Chadwick, P. (1986). Baccalaureate education and NCLEX: The causes of success. *Journal of Nursing Education, 25*(3), 94–101.

Yocum, C., & Scherubel, J. (1985). Selected pre-admission and academic correlates of success on state board examinations. *Journal of Nursing Education, 24*(6), 244–249.

11

The Failing Student: The Trials of Fulfilling One's Responsibility

Nurse educators are obligated by professional nursing standards, as well as the tenets of education, to graduate individuals qualified to engage in safe, effective nursing practice. This requires that nurse educators evaluate the clinical as well as the theoretical components of students' learning experiences, an idea that raises concern for many nurse educators. At what point does one conclude that adequate time has been provided for learning, and evaluation is appropriate? Evaluation represents the end point of a learning experience, but in the clinical setting, this point is more difficult to determine than in theory.

In addition to determining the appropriate point for evaluation, educators often are faced with the question of what to do when the student does not agree with the assignment of a grade, particularly a failing grade. Failure in a learning experience evokes a sense of personal failure, oftentimes for the nurse educator as well as for the student. This is exacerbated for the faculty person when the student receiving the grade appears to be surprised by, or angered by the failing grade. It is important for the educator to be aware of the appropriate steps that should be carried out to minimize the student's and the faculty member's feelings of helplessness during these times.

A failure can occur in the theoretical portion of a course, the clinical portion, or both. A theoretical failure generally is less painful for both the educator and the student because there is an established objective measure, the examination, by which all students can judge their progress or lack of it. In the clinical setting, however, the assignment of a grade even a grade of "pass" or "fail" for performance is based on a subjective assessment of behaviors, despite the existence of clearly written objectives. Several authors (Carpenito & Duespohl, 1985; Infante, 1985) have proposed ways to minimize the subjectivity of clinical evaluation, but no clear-cut solution to this problem has been found; therefore, it continues to plague clinical teachers.

Perhaps such concerns could be lessened by clearly articulating what evaluation is all about, when and how evaluation occurs, and who participates in the evaluation. Such an understanding is helpful in clarifying many issues related to evaluation.

PHASES OF EVALUATION

Two phases of evaluation predominate discussions of student evaluation. Educators currently use the terms *formative* and *summative* to describe the process of student evaluation. These terms were used originally by Scriven (1967) to describe program evaluation.

Formative Evaluation

Formative evaluation refers to the ongoing process of directing students during the learning experience. Students are apprised of strengths and weaknesses as they perform expected behaviors, and they are informed of their progress in meeting defined goals. Learners have the opportunity during this evaluative process to make mistakes, correct them, and explore alternative means of meeting prescribed goals. Ideally, during this phase of the evaluative process students are afforded the opportunity to make mistakes without being penalized.

In the classroom, formative evaluation of learning can be carried out through the use of unannounced, ungraded quizzes, or through ungraded out-of-class assignments. In clinical settings, the quality of daily care plans or students' responses to questions about laboratory tests, nursing care, or pathophysiology represent formative evaluation measures. These assessments allow the teacher to identify students' strengths and the work that will need to be completed to help the student meet preestablished clinical outcomes. Clinical instructors need

to share their assessments with students and suggest ways performance can be improved.

Summative Evaluation

Summative evaluation represents a judgment about student performance at the endpoint of a learning experience. During this phase, educators make judgments about students' abilities in meeting expected
goals at the end of experiences. Summative evaluation is based on the
expectation that formative evaluation has been carried out on a regular basis. It is, however, more than the total of formative evaluations
that have occurred during the course of a learning experience.

LINKING LEARNING OBJECTIVES
TO THE EVALUATION PROCESS

It should be apparent that learning and evaluation occur simultaneously; indeed, the two practices can be separated only artificially. The
key factor in the teaching-evaluation process, however, is to allow opportunities for learning and mistakes. Teachers should not hold students' poor judgment against them during the learning phase; instead,
the instructor should point out the problem, guide students in how to
deal with similar situations in the future, and reserve final judgment of
the students' abilities until later in the experience. Teachers must remain fair during observations of students (Carpenito, 1983), and they
must remember that students are feeling individuals who need to
have their strengths acknowledged. Students also need to be provided
with feedback during the formative phase of evaluation, thereby affording them the opportunity to grow and to be unsuccessful without
feeling that a situation is hopeless.

Students should be made aware of the purpose of evaluation and
that it will occur on a regular basis. If students are informed early of
the expectation that they be "on" all of the time, a different level of
preparation usually results. Students will arrive in the clinical and the
classroom setting prepared to demonstrate their knowledge.

In the classroom setting, the educator usually controls many of
the conditions that influence students' learning. Readings are assigned, lectures given, discussions directed, evaluation measures pre-

pared by the teacher, and evaluation intervals designated. In this way, there is tremendous responsibility on the educator to direct student learning. Depending on how the classroom milieu develops, the educator can assume more or less responsibility for how students in a particular classroom setting learn material. Some educators believe that it is their ultimate responsibility to impart all theoretical material through classroom lecture. Other teachers place all the responsibility for learning on the student and act only as "clearinghouses" to clarify misinterpreted or misunderstood material.

Between these two extremes are the educators who facilitate student learning through lecture-discussion, independent learning, and other creative approaches to teaching and learning. Responsibility for learning in this situation is shared. From these comments one might surmise that there are three distinct ways to impart material to be learned: teacher controlled, self-directed student learning, or both; in reality, any combination of these may be used given the simplicity or complexity of the material presented.

Clarify Learning Objectives

When preparing learning materials for the theoretical component of a course, it is important to state the learning objectives for the specific content area clearly. This will minimize student difficulty with evaluation and strengthen the evaluation process. Gronlund (1981) directs educators to develop examination questions that relate to the stated objectives of the learning experience. An example is as follows:

Objective: The student will identify the parts of an initial nursing assessment.

Question: During an initial nursing assessment, the nurse will carry out which of the following?
1. Hemoglobin
2. Urinalysis
3. Apical pulse
4. Enema

In the example cited, the students know what the performance expectation is, and teachers have an evaluation measure that is relevant and fair. Using Gronlund's (1981) suggestion, both educators and students are directed in the teaching-learning situation.

FAILING THE THEORY COMPONENT

When students fail an examination, certain steps can and should be carried out to reduce the enormity of the situation. First, instructors should meet with individual students to evaluate their perception of the failure and why they think it occurred. Students fail for a variety of reasons, such as the material is too complex, questions may be interpreted incorrectly, assigned readings may be too difficult, or students may have learning disabilities. Thus, it is important to determine what contributed to the failure and to counsel students to help them deal with those failures.

During individual conferences, educators should evaluate students' perceptions of their experience. Students may expedite this search for the reasons for failure by simply offering perceived causes. Some examples include inadequate preparation, personal problems, or lack of interest, and motivation. If students do not offer reasons, it will be necessary to work with them to identify causes. In a situation in which counseling, testing, or study skill experts are available, nurse educators may opt to set up an appointment to meet with these experts along with individual students. Such a joint meeting should offer all parties involved an opportunity to share their personal perspectives on the problem. If a meeting with a number of individuals is perceived by individual students to be threatening, nurse educators may wish to meet first with individual students, assess the reasons for their failures, and then send comments to the study and testing skill experts for inclusion in their evaluation.

Once the problem has been identified, students should be offered, by either the study and test skills expert or by nurse educators, ways to work toward remedying the situation. It then becomes each student's responsibility to improve the situation. Although educators can help students place a failure in perspective, it is important to remember that it is the student who must accept and deal with this event. Identifying the relationship of the failure to students' perceptions of themselves gives educators the ability to focus on the real issues at hand and move toward positive solutions.

When educators perceive that students are trying hard but still fail, they may begin to feel that somehow the failure is related to one's competence as a teacher. It is important to remember, however, that learning is the responsibility of each student. Teachers are responsible for guiding the learning experience and providing conditions that enhance learning. If the student still fails to learn, and ultimately fails, it is the student's failure, not the educator's. Despite this understanding, many teachers feel inadequate or helpless when students fail. To reduce feelings of inadequacy and helplessness in both students and teachers, nurse educators should consider several important steps that can be taken early in the learning situation to enhance the evaluation process.

WORKING WITH A FAILING STUDENT: MAXIMIZING RESOURCES

First, review the objectives of the unit to determine if they are clearly identified. Perhaps a review by a colleague with the same area of expertise or a curriculum coordinator could provide a valuable critique of the syllabus. In the event individuals available to review materials are not experts in the field, outside consultation may be needed. Such services are available through academic support networks, testing centers, or accrediting organizations.

In addition to the critique of the objectives, the readings suggested and the assignments required should be evaluated to determine whether or not they are adequate and relevant in helping students complete the objectives. It also may be helpful to videotape some class sessions and review the tapes to determine whether the information provided and the teaching strategies used are sufficient to help students complete all of the learning objectives. Ideally, the use of individuals who are unfamiliar with the subject matter will be most valuable in this analysis because they can offer an accurate evaluation of the completeness of the materials as they relate to the objectives.

Nurse educators also should evaluate whether the examination questions can be answered from the materials presented. Answers to the examination questions should be documented from the sources the students were directed to use to achieve the objectives. This is not meant to suggest that only printed materials are acceptable references for examination questions. If a lecture, film, or presentation is required material for a specific content area, then it is suitable to use this material in the development of examination questions. It is important, however, to avoid using anecdotal experiences drawn from the clinical setting in which all students were not present. Thus, the key to using materials not available in print form as the basis of examination questions is their relationship to the stated objectives and their availability to all students.

Once it has been established that appropriate conditions exist that give all students the opportunity to meet the objectives, educators should offer students who fail an examination a chance to review relevant materials. A private meeting between instructors and individual students is the most effective way to review course materials and the examination. This provides educators with the opportunity to assess students' difficulties on a one-to-one basis and gives students the feeling that teachers care about them. It also may be helpful to schedule a group test review, but teachers should be aware that the use of this format alone limits the ability to assess individual student difficulties.

In the case of examination failure, specific helpful hints for improving performance, as well as a strong vote of confidence for the student's future performance should be given. Conversely, course failure may necessitate assisting the student in defining new goals or alternative ways to meet the unattained goal. If the instructor evaluating the student does not feel comfortable in assisting the student to redefine goals, then refer the student to an appropriate resource, such as a faculty adviser or program director.

The referral of a student to a support system is important. Frequently overlooked, however, is the educator's need for support. It is vitally important for nurse educators to seek support systems for themselves. Operating in a vacuum will intensify feelings of failure or self-righteousness. In either case, the educator is in a situation in which perspective on the failure may be lost. Using peer networks can help keep the experience in perspective.

After nurse educators have reviewed the learning and evaluation materials, felt satisfied that they were appropriate, and met with the students who performed poorly or referred them to appropriate experts, they can be certain that their responsibilities have been met. Novice educators have more difficulty than senior teachers acknowledging and accepting that the teacher is expert, and because of their expertise, they have the right to make decisions regarding the appropriateness of materials.

When admitted to an institution, student success is not guaranteed. The educator may do well to remember that although she or he facilitates learning, the onus for fulfillment of educational goals is on the student. The student must be goal directed and motivated to complete the program of study. When difficulties arise, educators should provide appropriate support and guidance, and students must accept responsibility and move forward.

FAILING THE CLINICAL COMPONENT

In the clinical setting, the ability to evaluate the student in an objective manner is much more difficult. Although clinical goals are offered verbally or in writing before most clinical experiences, the interpretation of success or failure in meeting those goals is largely at the discretion of the clinical teacher. Infante (1985) describes the part the word *value* holds in the word *evaluation*.

> The value system of the evaluator is inadvertently contained in the methods selected and the processes instituted to make the judgments. So by its very nature, the evaluation process is heavily laden with subjectivity. (p. 149)

Primarily for this reason, clinical failure represents a more painful experience for both students and educators, forcing educators to continually reevaluate their own values when clinical failure of one of their students becomes a possibility or a reality.

To minimize some of the trauma of this experience, educators should follow through with many of the same steps described in the treatment of theoretical failures. There should be explicit objectives that are available to students early in the learning experience, and these objectives should be clearly stated and attainable for the given level of student. Clinical educators must provide students with experiences that will help them meet the objectives. For instance, an objective such as "The student will provide preoperative teaching to an open-heart patient" may not be attainable by every student if some of the students are placed on medical units or if special opportunities for this type of experience are not made available.

In addition to explicitly stating the objectives, students must be provided with feedback regarding the quality of their performance. This creates a dilemma for some clinical educators, namely at what point is learning expected to have occurred and can evaluation be carried out fairly? As described earlier, there are two types of evaluation, formative and summative. In the clinical setting, formative evaluation occurs during the learning of new skills or procedures. Summative evaluation occurs at the end of a learning experience, which can be at mid-term or at the end of a semester, depending on the structure of the program.

Some faculty groups opt to implement summative clinical evaluation by assigning specific evaluation days that occur at specific points during a learning experience. Using this model, the educator evaluates how the student meets the goals of the clinical aspects of the course on the designated evaluation day(s) and disregards the student's "up and downs" that occurred during previous clinical days. This places a tremendous stress on some students to perform on evaluation day(s). Conversely, it establishes an environment that permits errors during the learning process without penalty.

Other educators prefer a more continuous evaluation method, that is, a regular observation of abilities with ongoing critique throughout the learning experience, all of which is included in the end-point evaluation. An example of this method is the evaluation of surgical asepsis each time a student carries it out. When this evaluative model is used, students report they are never given credit for proficiency and feel the constant pressure of evaluation. Sharing with students the reality that nurses must always be "on" may help to deflate some of the anxiety experienced. The advantage of this method is that students are provided with the opportunity to develop their skills and be evaluated on an ongoing basis rather than having the total grade for their clinical experience based on a single concentrated evaluation.

Another way of evaluating involves the critique of only the objective designated for the day or week of clinical. This approach has its own problems given that it may be impossible to provide every student with an experience to meet a stated objective during a specific period. One of the advantages, however, is that it keeps students and faculty focused on specific material to be evaluated during a particular period. It also provides a structure that has the possibility of maximizing performance of expected behaviors as they relate to classroom instruction.

Regardless of the approach used for clinical evaluation, most educators would agree that motor skills are the easiest to evaluate. Even this seemingly clear-cut area is fraught with controversy, however. Some teachers would argue that a student either can or cannot perform a skill. Others contend that there are levels of performance and question whether students who take 30 minutes to change a dressing without any break in technique should receive the same passing grade as the student who carries out the procedure in 5 minutes but admittedly forgets to open the dressings before donning sterile gloves. To remedy this situation, some educators have developed lengthy evaluation measures describing the appropriate steps with time limits and verbal responses expected for each and every skill. This may be an appropriate strategy in the evaluation of motor skills, but is less useful in the evaluation of cognitive and affective skills.

An objective such as "the student will demonstrate effective organization of work habits" is a difficult objective to evaluate. The question needs to be asked, according to what standard is the effectiveness of the work judged? What specific behaviors is the educator assessing? Will each clinical teacher have the same criteria to judge this objective?

FLEXIBILITY IN THE EVALUATIVE PROCESS

How do clinical educators deal with students who do not meet the clinical objectives and fail the clinical portion of the course knowing that these students may have to repeat the entire course and be delayed in achieving their career goal for a year or more? How does the clinical teacher uphold standards of practice and still allow students learning time?

Many elements related to clinical evaluation of students who do not perform at expected levels are illustrated in the letter presented at the beginning of this unit. As an example, the student presented in the letter appears to be working at her optimum. At the bedside, however, she is "awkward and disorganized"; she does not demonstrate a bedside manner that provides the client with even a minimal confidence level in her abilities; she has repeatedly been sent back to the skills laboratory to relearn and practice techniques, each time returning with similar problems; redemonstration of skills in the clinical area are accurate only about 30% of the time. How would the clinical educator handle this situation to minimize the uneasiness felt by both teacher and student during the assignment of a failing grade?

First and foremost, a referral to tutoring early is an excellent action. The student's motor skills were lacking as were her verbal abilities, and they need to be assessed by an expert. Some of the problem may be related to her command of the English language, but given the available information, a complete assessment is indicated. Tutors enhance the student's opportunities to improve and remove some of the burden for problem identification from the nurse educator.

The principles of teaching and learning theory suggest the importance of the learner feeling successful at new experiences. If this is not possible because of overall poor performance, it is critical to separate the failure at a skill from the failure as a person (Turkett, 1987). Students sometimes come to a new learning situation feeling unsuccessful as people, and any criticism of their performance further exacerbates their feelings of insecurity. It is valuable, when this type of situation is identified, for teachers to be sensitive to how they interact with such students and to refer them for counseling. Individuals need to believe they are successful people to feel successful when faced with a failing experience. Nurse educators have a responsibility to be aware of the difference. Students may fail at a particular learning experience, but this does not mean that they are unsuccessful as individuals. Nurse educators can reduce these feelings by pointing out the successes that individual students have experienced in other areas. A positive approach will enhance students' perspectives on their own development.

When approaching students about unsuccessful clinical behaviors, remember always to do so privately, not in front of others. Students should be made aware of unacceptable performances as soon as possible after they occur and be offered ways in which the expected behaviors can be carried out successfully. The clinical teacher may need to direct the student to return to the skills laboratory or prepare a care plan or paper to enrich learning.

When students return to the clinical area after remediation, they should be given the opportunity to perform the previously failed skill. A vote of confidence from the instructor will be beneficial for most students.

If the behavior is still below acceptable standards after a second attempt, instructors should again carry out the previously described process. They should be aware of the fact that with each unsuccessful attempt at a behavior, the student's anxiety level heightens, which may further impede performance. If this is obviously occurring, an evaluation by another faculty member may be a beneficial course of action to follow. Each situation will need to be evaluated individually by faculty members to decide whether this is a viable option for students.

Additionally, it is important to provide students with comprehensive evaluations of overall performance at designated points. During these evaluation conferences, as stated earlier, educators should point out students' strengths and weaknesses and offer specific ways to improve those weaknesses. Student advisers should also be apprised of the problems and deficiencies of their advisees as should any other person or department on campus who is working with specific students to improve their shortcomings.

If students have been informed throughout the clinical experience of their deficiencies and have been given the opportunity to improve, followed by the occasion to demonstrate the deficient behaviors again, educators have fulfilled their responsibilities to students. If students verbalize discontent with the evaluation, the discussion should always be refocused on what part individual students played in failing to meet the educational objectives for the learning experience. Similar to the theoretical failure discussed earlier, this may be the time to reevaluate long-term plans and goals.

The responsibility for failing a course is the student's. If nurse educators have provided appropriate opportunities for learning, then they have adequately carried out their responsibilities, and there is no need to feel guilty about the outcome.

In addition to sharing students' deficiencies with them, nurse educators should document carefully, being certain to separate facts from judgmental statements. Each deficient behavior should be documented along with the actions prescribed by the teacher to correct the problem. At the initial identification of deficiencies, it is useful to develop a written contract with students that identifies their plans for meeting the required objective. This procedure is a safeguard for both educators and students, and the documentation serves as a point of reference for future conferences.

The assignment of a failing grade to any student is a difficult task for most faculty members. The negative feelings evoked can be alleviated, however, if educators remember that they are not failures themselves. The student's failure is the failure of *one* experience; regardless of how much the educator would like to change the situation, it remains the student's dilemma. To maintain the standards of the nursing profession, there must be a commitment to the development and perpetuation of excellence. Keeping this goal in mind should provide solace to educators in situations in which a student failure appears imminent.

One other area deserves discussion. When a student is failing clinically, other students frequently receive less guidance than they may need. Educators supervising a clinical group must remain cognizant of this fact. Students who perform poorly must be removed from the clinical area in which they are not prepared to function so that educators can be resources to all other students. If teachers are too distracted by a student who is performing poorly, the needs of the entire group may not be being met, and other students may not receive the learning experiences they deserve. Faculty should identify minimum competencies that are required to function in the clinical setting. If certain students are unable to perform these competencies, then they should be removed immediately from the clinical area until their deficient skills have been found to be satisfactory in a setting other than the clinical site.

SUMMARY

The failure of any experience is threatening for most individuals. To minimize the problems inherent in theoretical or clinical failures, nurse educators need to create an environment of acceptance and understanding. Although most students have a difficult time acknowledging it, failure actually provides an opportunity to grow and develop. A failed clinical or theoretical experience may merely represent a lack of development at a certain point in time; it does not necessarily mean that the student will never be a nurse. The goal can be reached if both educators and students remember that time and effort can improve most situations. Educators are the experts and for this reason are required to set the standards for the future. It is an awesome responsibility, but one nurse educators must accept when they choose to practice in the teaching role.

REFERENCES

Carpenito, L. S. (1983). The failing or unsatisfactory student. *Nurse Educator*, 8(4), 32–33.

Carpenito, L. S., & Duespohl, T. A. (1985). *A guide to effective clinical education* (2nd ed.). Rockville, MD: Aspen.

Gronlund, N. E. (1981). *Measurement and evaluation in teaching* (4th ed.). New York: MacMillan.

Infante, M. S. (1985). *The clinical laboratory in nursing education* (2nd ed.). New York: Wiley.

Scriven, M. (1967). *The methodology of evaluation* (AERA Monograph Series in Curriculum Evaluation No. 1). Chicago: Rand McNally.

Turkett, S. (1987). Let's take the "i" out of failure. *Journal of Nursing Education*, 26(6), 246–247.

12

The Teacher's Responsibility for Protecting the Rights of Students and Patients

When the word *legal* enters a conversation it frequently evokes a sense of concern and, in many cases, feelings of dread. If one looks at the legal aspects of teaching as one of the essential considerations of the role of teacher, however, the educator can approach this aspect with confidence and objectivity. Today's educators need not practice from a defensive posture when it comes to either their own or students' legal rights. Knowing each other's rights is a way of protecting and enhancing that which is due an individual.

Since the civil rights marches of the 1960s, the people of the United States have developed a new consciousness about their legitimate right to be protected from discrimination. The issue of discrimination has highlighted individuals' due process rights. It is the intent of this chapter to closely examine the legal rights of individuals involved in the teaching-learning situation and how they are protected by specific amendments to the Constitution.

When individuals enter hospitals they have a right to expect that they will be taken care of by the health care staff and will be treated courteously during their stay. These rights have been described in detail by both the NLN in their statement of *Nursing's Role in Patients' Rights* (1977) and by the American Hospital Association (1972) in their document entitled, *A Patient's Bill of Rights*.

Similarly, students engaged in the teaching-learning situation have a right to expect that their participation in the experience will produce some beneficial outcome. They also have the right to expect that they will be treated fairly as they seek to achieve a particular educational goal (*Student Bill of Rights*, 1975).

In addition to students' rights in the teaching-learning situation, faculty members and agencies that participate in student learning experiences also have rights; faculty members have the right to pursue teaching responsibilities without undue restrictions by the college or university; and health care agencies have the right to expect that the care of clients will be a prime concern during the teaching situation. Given all of these individual rights, how can nursing educators begin to exercise their responsibilities in the classroom and clinical setting? How does an educator provide for or enhance student learning in the classroom while attending to students' rights?

STUDENTS' RIGHTS

The umbrella concept under which discussions of students' rights occurs is that rights of individuals do not stand in isolation; instead they are accompanied by responsibilities. In fact, whenever individuals claim violation of their rights, an inquiry is required to determine the nature of the responsibilities of the individual or organization who is said to have violated their rights. For instance, students cannot claim that their rights are violated if a college or university refuses to provide them with transportation to a school athletic function to be a spectator. The institution does not have a responsibility to provide transportation to spectators of sporting events, so no right has been violated.

In contrast, a student who is not provided some evaluation measure for a course taken for credit because the instructor chooses not to give any has experienced violation of a right. Students have a right to expect evaluative feedback in their work, and faculty members have the responsibility to provide evaluation criteria for courses that are offered for credit. Faculty members cannot arbitrarily decide not to submit evaluations.

Students' Rights in the Classroom

It is not unusual for faculty members to encounter students who fail an examination or term paper assignment. Using this as an example, the issue of students' rights in the classroom and faculty member's responsibilities with respect to these rights can be examined.

Before beginning a discussion of student failure, it is important to point out that the court "has rejected the notion that access to higher education is a fundamental right" (Golden, 1981–1982, p. 496). In Keyes v. Sawyer (1973), a complex case in which a student, after receiving two failing grades and being unsuccessful in having the grades changed published libelous statements about the professors and was subsequently dismissed, appealed to the courts to render a decision providing for reinstatement. In this case, Keyes requested that the court direct the professors to change his grades claiming that his "failure to be readmitted to the institution was a violation of the Civil Rights Act [of 1871] on the grounds that he had a constitutional right to a public education" (Toombs & DiBiase, 1974, p. 359). The Court, however, in rendering a decision stated that Keyes "had no constitutional right to education but he had a constitutional right to equal opportunity to partake of public education offered by the state" (Toombs & DiBiase, 1974, p. 359). These statements affirm that the courts have determined individuals do not have a property or liberty interest at stake when they are dismissed from public colleges or universities (Golden, 1981–1982). This information should be of help to educators in their interactions with students, particularly when the prospect of failure or dismissal becomes a reality.

What should educators do specifically to fulfill their teaching responsibilities while remaining cognizant of students' rights? Before the initiation of any course, students have the right to know what the course description is, what the objectives are, what the expectations of the course are, and what the evaluation measures are. If instructors make this information available during the first class, they already have a head start in fulfilling their responsibilities and therefore protecting students' rights.

After an examination is given or a paper is handed in, the student has a right to expect that the examination or paper is corrected and returned within a time frame that would provide the student with an opportunity to improve performance prior to completion of the course. Marx (1984) states the following:

The more notice a student has of the academic performance expected of him, and the more notice a student has of his impending failure while there is yet time to meet the expectation, the less formal any subsequent hearing on the consequences of the failure needs to be. (p. 56)

A question may arise related to what the educator should do if only one paper or one examination is given for the entire course, and the student fails. This situation puts both the educator and the student in a precarious position. It is extremely difficult to measure students progress toward some learning outcome if only one grade is available. Students should be able to be unsuccessful in parts of learning experiences without the consequence being failure of the course.

If students have the criteria for successful completion of the course, and they fail a paper or an examination, then the students have the responsibility to seek out ways of improving performance in the course. Faculty need not fear retaliation for assigning a failing grade. In fact, "Courts have been consistent in their support of teachers and their [teachers] authority to award grades to students and have spoken to this issue on numerous occasions" (Walden & Gamble, 1985, pp. 610–611). Thus, if a failing grade is justified, nurse educators should feel comfortable assigning it. To date, the courts have not become involved in grade awards. The concern of the legal system has not been the grade but rather whether student rights have been violated.

In support of students, nursing faculties have been exemplary in their advocacy for students through the initiation of support mechanisms, such as exam reviews and tutoring. These types of supports are not required by the legal system but certainly enhance students' perceptions of their value and self-worth. When faculty take time to provide an extra measure of assistance, students receive a message that they are valued, and their success in the course is important to faculty members. This type of caring and concern is often enough to help students regain confidence in their ability to meet course expectations and, in fact, help them to succeed.

If the occasion arises and students fail despite their best efforts, the failures need to be accepted as the individual student's. Nursing faculty cannot bear the burden of responsibility for those who are unable to complete the program of study. Nursing curricula demand students use their intellectual abilities fully and demonstrate a level of commitment. If either of these qualities are deficient, nursing educators must accept that it is not their fault.

In a time of great demand for students, it is hoped that admission criteria are maintained since these criteria are developed based on sound knowledge of the minimal requirements for success. When educational institutions do not establish criteria by which to admit students or when they become lax about those criteria, then the difficulty for both the faculty and the student when failure occurs is greater. A disservice is done to the student who is admitted to a nursing program with low-level abilities because nursing curricula are intense and rigorous, requiring both academic ability and commitment.

Due Process

When a student fails and perceives that the educator has in some way been unfair in assigning a clinical or theoretical grade, a grievance may be initiated. Most colleges and universities have grievance procedures outlined in the college catalog or student handbook, and most such procedures are based on the rights of individuals that are protected by the fourteenth amendment to the Constitution. It is important for educators to be familiar with the college or university's student grievance policy and knowledgeable about what warrants grievance procedures. Additionally, faculty members should become familiar with what their role in the grievance procedure may be.

The courts of this country have generally held that academic matters do not require the same type of due process procedure as disciplinary matters. Academic matters generally include knowledge or skills required by a program of study. Disciplinary matters relate to those violations of institutional codes of conduct and would include, but not be limited to, plagiarism or violation of visitation rules. Students who face dismissal for disciplinary reasons are required by law to have a more elaborate due process procedure accorded them than those facing academic dismissal.

Grievance procedures outlined in school materials are basically due process procedures developed specifically for a particular university or college. The procedures outlined usually identify the types of situations that warrant a due process or grievance hearing, the levels of hearing and appeal, the time factors to be upheld in the process, and the number and constituency of the individuals who are charged with reviewing the grievance. Limandri (1981); Logsdon, Lacefield, and Clark (1979); Majorowicz (1986); and Miller (1982) have written about specific grievance policies developed within their organizations to handle academic grievances; these examples may be helpful to nurse educators seeking to develop a grievance procedure.

Student Responsibilities for Initiation of a Grievance

When a student opts to initiate a court proceeding to remedy a dismissal from a program or institution, the student must fulfill several requirements. First, the student must be able to demonstrate that he or she has completely exhausted the appropriate channels within the college or university. The student must also be able to prove that a property or liberty interest has been violated. The "Supreme Court has consistently found a property right to exist where . . . statutory entitlement has been created" (Golden, 1981–1982, p. 496). Statutory entitlement means that individuals are entitled to a particular interest based on state laws, rules, or understandings. The Supreme Court has also held that individuals have property rights based on custom or institutional policy. For example, a student who maintains satisfactory academic standing and pays required fees has a valid property right to graduate based on previous students' experiences in a particular institution. In some instances students have brought charges against colleges and universities based on their perception that attendance at a particular institution represents a property right and that subsequent dismissal violates this right. Generally speaking, the courts have not accepted the student's right to an education as a property right at the postsecondary level. Mere attendance at an institution of higher learning does not represent a property right. Satisfactory academic performance, maintenance of conduct expected by the institution, and payment of fees generally establishes a property right.

In terms of student's liberty interests, the Supreme Court has included the student's right to his or her reputation, honor, and integrity. As an illustration, a college cannot publicly announce a student's violations of academic or disciplinary matters without providing the individual due process.

Faculty Protection of Students' Due Process Rights

Within the college or university system, it becomes extremely important for educators to be aware of the institutional policies governing students' rights to due process. As stated earlier, it is important also that nurse educators be aware of what activities are protected under the due process guidelines within the institution. Once these are known, then the faculty member can act appropriately when an incident arises necessitating exercise of these rights.

To prepare for the unlikely event that legal claims against the department or institution are brought, nursing faculty should provide a few safeguards for themselves and their students. First, they should review the college or university policy to ascertain whether or not there is a statement that reflects the student's rights at the department level. If there is such a statement, is it understood by everyone? In addition, how is the statement implemented at the department level? If no guidelines are available within the department they should be developed, approved by the appropriate body, and promulgated widely.

Second, a mechanism should exist to provide support for both the student and the educator in the event a due process hearing is initiated, because the course of a due process hearing can be difficult for all of the parties involved. By having a mechanism in place before the procedure, individuals involved can be assisted in the preparation, implemention, and completion of due process activities.

Third, a regular cycle of orientation and in-service education to new and existing faculty should be provided to keep them fully apprised of the procedure and any changes in the law. As stated earlier, the courts have chosen not to become involved in academic matters to date. When a case is brought to court regarding a violation of property or liberty interests, specifically as they relate to academic matters within public colleges and universities, the courts generally have only evaluated whether or not due process procedures have been met. As stated earlier, the courts have not required the same degree of due process in academic matters.

Marx (1984) outlined the steps to be taken in academic dismissal procedures to protect the educator and institution from claims. First, institutions should publish expected standards for student conduct at the institution and have them available for review.

Second, every student should be provided an orientation session in which the standards are offered. Third, students who are in academic jeopardy should be informed of such an evaluation in time for corrective measures to be taken on the part of the student to improve the performance.

Fourth, before dismissal every student should have the opportunity to be heard. This opportunity should occur in an informal manner similar to a counseling session. The reason for this hearing is so the student is able to present his or her perceptions of the reason why dismissal should not occur. Marx (1984) recommends that the hearing occur before a dean or dean designee, someone other than the professor giving the dismissal notice. He also suggests that the outcome of the decision be written and shared with the student.

Finally a mechanism should be in place for an appeal process. In general, the courts have not required this to be a lengthy procedure. Reversal of academic dismissal proceedings has occurred only when the courts have found the institutions to have acted in an arbitrary or capricious fashion, that is, without reason or in sudden and unpredictable ways. An example of this would be a situation in which senior nursing students are offered the opportunity to select their own clinical sites but one person is told that the faculty member will decide where she is to go. This kind of action would be considered arbitrary and capricious on the part of the faculty member.

Due Process in Clinical Settings

To safeguard the position of the clinical instructor in determining student performance outcomes, faculty would be served well by instituting similar procedures for clinical failures. It is important to state, however, that nursing academicians have been arduous in their pursuit of quantifiable and measurable student learning outcomes in the clinical arena. The courts have not been as arduous in their interpretation of measurable outcomes. The Board of Curators of University of Missouri v. Horowitz (1978) case clearly identified that medical professionals have the right to determine what is acceptable medical protocol in the exercise of physician-patient relations. In this case, Horowitz was dismissed from medical school "because of clinical performance, where she was found to have deficiencies in relations with faculty and others and personal habits considered not appropriate for clinical practice" (Arkin, 1985, p. 2463) despite successful academic performance in the classroom.

Similar to Horwitz (1978), nursing faculty might find if tested in court that their perceptions of unacceptable professional nursing behavior would stand and would not require a lengthy list of activities or objectives. In essence, the courts have afforded professionals the freedom and the responsibility to set their own academic standards based on their expertise.

PATIENT CARE AND FACULTY RESPONSIBILITY

Repeatedly, faculty verbalize concerns when asked what they perceive to be their legal responsibility in the clinical setting, and many make statements that reflect beliefs that "students practice on my license." Thus, it is important to examine the role of faculty in the assignment and care of patients during the clinical learning laboratory experience.

Faculty members have the responsibility for providing students with experiences for which they have received appropriate instruction. Given that students have learned about caring for clients in particular situations, they do *not* practice on nurse educators' licenses. In fact, students are held directly accountable—in a court of law—for any activity that they carry out, just as faculty members are held accountable for activities that they initiate. When students feel ill prepared or unable to carry out a procedure, it is their responsibility to inform faculty members. Likewise, graduate nurses have the responsibility to inform their supervisors if they have an inadequate knowledge base to carry out particular activities.

Nursing educators should choose student assignments carefully, attending to the student's knowledge base and the objectives of the course. Clinical instructors have a responsibility, then, to teach students in the clinical area, to supervise the activities of students during the experience, and to evaluate students' performance and give prompt, constructive, objective feedback. Faculty can be held accountable if students cause harm to patients while carrying out assignments given to them by faculty for which they are inadequately prepared. Generally speaking, however, the responsibility for student error in the clinical area is always the student's. Nevertheless, faculty members do have the obligation to see that the assignments are appropriate, given the student's knowledge base and preparation. Knowingly allowing a student to carry out a procedure for which no instruction has been provided is inviting danger.

There will be occasions when students and graduates have to carry out procedures for which no specific instruction has occurred. When this situation arises, the practitioners must be provided with the resources to learn about the procedure. This can occur through reading about the procedure and then being guided by an RN or faculty member in carrying it out. Opportunitites to provide experiences in all the activities that a nurse may ever encounter in her professional career is impossible. The important considerations if a court case results are (a) whether the nurse or student nurse sought out the knowledge needed; (b) whether the activity was permissible under the Nurse Practice Act in the state in which the litigation is occurring; and (c) whether the nurse or student nurse acted in a prudent manner in the particular situation.

Regardless of the circumstance, if a patient is injured while under the care of a student, the hospital, the staff nurse whose patient assignment is used for the learning experience, his or her immediate supervisor, the attending physician, the clinical instructor, and the student usually would all be named in the suit. As individual lines of responsibility and accountability are explored, those individuals who acted appropriately would be dropped from the suit. Although clinical faculty most likely would not be held accountable for flagrant actions of students, such as administering an intramuscular injection without prior instruction, clinical instructors would have to give testimony to their knowledge of the students' competence levels.

SUMMARY

In conclusion, legal aspects of the faculty role are multifaceted, and all rights are accompanied by responsibilities. Faculty members would be wise to learn as much as possible about all parts of the faculty role before assuming responsibility for any assignment. It is important to understand that as professionals, nursing educators will be held accountable for those activities for which they accept responsibility.

REFERENCES

A patient's bill of rights. (1972). Chicago: American Hospital Association.

Arkin, H. R. (1985). Academic dismissal: Due process. *JAMA, 254*(17), 2463–2466.

Board of Curators of University of Missouri v. Horwitz, 435 U.S. 78 (1978).

Golden, E. J. (1981–1982). College student dismissals and the Eldridge factors: What process is due? *Journal of College and University Law, 8*(4), 495–509.

Keys v. Sawyer, 353 F. Supp. 936 (1973).

Limandri, B. J. (1981). Academic procedural due process for students in the health professions. *Journal of Nursing Education, 20*(2), 9–18.

Logsdon, J. B., Lacefield, P. K., & Clark, M. J. (1979). The development of an academic grievance procedure. *Nursing Outlook, 27*(3), 184–190.

Majorowicz, K. (1986). Clinical grades and the grievance process. *Nurse Educator, 11*(2), 36–40.

Marx, C. A. (1984). Horowitz: A defense point of view. *Journal of Law & Education, 13*(1), 51–58.

Miller, P. (1982). Student grade appeals — Procedure and process. *Journal of Nursing Education, 21*(6), 34–38.

Nursing's role in patients' rights (1977). New York: National League for Nursing.

Student bill of rights (1975). New York: National Student Nurses' Association.

Toombs, W., & DiBiase, E. (1974). College rules and court decisions: Notes on student dismissals. *Journal of College and University Law, 2*(4), 355–368.

Walden, J. C., & Gamble, L. R. (1985). Student promotion and retention policies and legal considerations. *Journal of Law and Education, 14*(4), 609–623.

UNIT V
Faculty Evaluation

LETTERS

Dear Terry,

This will probably be one of my shorter letters. I've been very busy at school trying to tie up loose ends as another year comes to a close. It is hard to believe how fast semesters go by. To show you just how fast it does go, guess who was asked to mentor one of next year's new faculty? Yup! Me! Seems that not so long ago, I was a novice myself and some "old timer" was "showing me the ropes!"

In sitting down to put together an information packet for the new faculty member, I realized that materials were somewhat sketchy in one area: faculty evaluation. What a dreaded two words. I remember the first year I was here and I needed to be evaluated by the dean of faculty, the chairperson of the department, the level coordinator, and a colleague of my choosing. I can still recall all too vividly the anxiety that the whole experience caused. Today, I guess I just look at it as one more aspect of being a faculty member.

I still wonder now, as I wondered then, what faculty evaluation really is all about. Who are these people who hold the destiny of my career in the ink of their pens? Why do we do it? I know on an intellectual level why we do it, but at some deeper level I wonder what part it plays in the overall scenario of faculty careers. A great deal of emphasis is placed on student, faculty, and administrative ratings of faculty. Is a faculty member who sits in my class for one session really getting a true picture of my teaching skills? Are the students who evaluate my clinical teaching skills truly knowledgeable about all of the components of clinical education? Does my attendance at conferences and the papers I present really tell you about my scholarship? Obviously some tenure committees think so. All of the parts of the evaluation process seem to add up to such a small part of what I do and how I do it.

Another question that crosses my mind regularly is: How can my colleagues outside of nursing (e.g., the dean of faculty) really understand all of the components of a nursing faculty role? For example, the biology faculty have repeatedly complained about the nursing faculty work load. They equate biology lab with the hospital time, not knowing how incredibly different the two situations are. For one thing, I never get a clinical lab assistant! I also need to prepare for and evaluate that experience so differently. Needless to say, if the biology faculty sees a student cut the aorta during dissection of the fetal pig, little harm is done. From the nursing perspective, if I miss a student's miscalculation of a heparin dose and the patient receives three times the prescribed dose, the consequences are potentially fatal. Even a non-health care person can see the obvious differences in the gravity of these two situations. Yet despite these and other differences, everyone is evaluated in the same way, using the same criteria.

I am hopeful that you can offer some of your useful, insightful information. What would I do without you? You have been such a wonderful friend. How will I ever be able to repay you for all of your support?

DEAR HELEN,

Time does fly, doesn't it?! It doesn't take long for the novice to become the expert once new novices come on board.

I am always fascinated by the reactions of faculty members to the whole process of—indeed, the mere *thought* of—being evaluated. Nursing faculty members are probably *the* most precise and conscientious faculty on campus; but when we contemplate our own evaluation, our knees get weak.

As faculty members, we evaluate everything and continually! We evaluate students in the classroom and clinical areas. We give tests, grade papers and nursing care plans, assess students' contributions to class discussions, and observe and judge students' clinical performance. At the end of each semester, we ask students to evaluate the course, the teachers, the clinical agencies used, the films they saw, the textbooks they used, etc. We make careful judgments about clinical learning environments to determine their appropriateness for future use. We determine the effectiveness of our teaching strategies and our tests. We decide on the usefulness of the textbook we used and constantly search for new and better books. We are educated and socialized to use the nursing process, which includes a strong evaluation component, and we are all too keenly aware of the evaluations we do and undergo as part of our accreditation review.

One would think with all this exposure to, involvement in and (supposed) valuing of the evaluation process, we wouldn't be so frightened of it. I suppose when it is each of us personally who is being scrutinized and judged, however, we become particularly aware of the subjective nature of such evaluations and the impact they can have on our careers.

Perhaps some of the concerns faculty express over being evaluated are exactly the same we struggle with when evaluating students in the clinical area. Evaluations such as these *are* subjective. There is no way around that, and the sooner we can accept that and live with it, the quicker we can move on to gaining from the evaluation process.

Even when the criteria for evaluation are clear, they are subject to a variety of interpretations, and the judgments made can be influenced by factors that are (theoretically) unrelated. Perhaps one of the things that might make faculty feel more comfortable with being judged is to seek clarification from those doing the evaluation about their interpretation of the criteria, and to do this well in advance of when the evaluation will be completed. Just as faculty members tell students to ask at the beginning of the semester for interpretation of course objectives, they should ask the same kind of question about their evaluative criteria from the appropriate persons.

Faculty also should seek clarification about who will do the various parts of the evaluation, how data will be collected, who will review the material submitted, and what will be done with the evaluations after they are written. In a school or college of nursing, the course or level leader or the associate dean for Undergraduate Nursing Studies may do some aspects of the evaluation; in a department of nursing, the chairperson may do the entire evaluation; and in some structures, the only data filed are self-evaluation reports. It is important to know who will do your evaluation and what data will be used to make judgments.

Student evaluations of teachers is a significant aspect of faculty evaluations. Peer reviews also may be included as well as evaluations from committee chairpersons with whom you have worked, staff in the clinical agencies where you affiliate with students, and yourself. Faculty should have the right to review any of these materials before they are submitted to the dean or chairperson so any questionable areas can be answered or any points of concern addressed. The data being used to make judgments about a faculty member's effectiveness should not be kept secret from the person being evaluated!

One of the things that faculty often do not realize, however, is that one accomplishment in a given academic year is "rewarded" for that year but does not "count" in succeeding years. For example, an article published in January 1985 would be recognized as an accomplishment in your 1984–1985 evaluation, but in succeeding years, you will be expected to continue to publish new material. Faculty sometimes think once they have published an article, made a professional presentation, or served on a committee it ought to be enough to last them for the remainder of their academic careers. You know, of course, this is not the way the system works because academics are expected to continue to make significant contributions to their departments or schools as well as to their professions. When faculty members fail to continue to make such contributions, they may not be evaluated very positively.

We've discussed many times before the fact that faculty members have many roles to play and many responsibilities to fulfill. When it comes time for evaluation, they are judged on their performance and contributions in each of those areas. Perhaps one of the disservices faculty members do to themselves and to each other, however, is to set up the expectation that each person will excel in *each* of those areas *all* the time. That, as you well know, is impossible.

The criteria and mechanisms used for faculty evaluations need to recognize the impossibility of faculty being supermen or superwomen. In my opinion, the evaluation process also needs to take into consideration the uniqueness of each discipline. In some fields, it is almost impossible to get an article published in a refereed journal, whereas in other disciplines, it in not as difficult. In some disciplines (such as biology), it is easier to combine laboratory research activities with one's teaching assignment, whereas in other areas (like nursing) one must make a special effort to do laboratory or clinical research. In other fields (like history), the nature of the teaching assignment is relatively stable, whereas in others (like nursing) a faculty member must be engaged in classroom, laboratory, and clinical instruction, each of which requires a different set of skills and abilities. If these differences were recognized somehow in the faculty evaluation process, faculty might be less concerned about the whole area and more confident about what they *are* achieving than worried about what they are *not* achieving.

You have raised some excellent questions about the validity of peer evaluations, the value of being evaluated by members of a discipline other than your own, and the objectivity of student evaluations of teaching. These are very important questions to raise and ones that deserve much discussion. Unfortunately, I don't think these issues can be addressed adequately through a letter, so let's plan to meet to talk about them in the not-too-distant future. Suffice it to say I believe that if the purpose of the evaluation is made very clear to the person doing the appraisal as well as the person being evaluated, any of these concerns soon become less important than they had seemed initially. Perhaps it is the whole question of purpose . . . Why do we do faculty evaluations in the first place? . . . that is the most significant and the most troublesome.

It seems to me the most important reason for conducting any evaluation is to give feedback regarding strengths and the areas that need improvement. The ultimate purpose of this is to enhance the product or service being delivered.

In educational jargon, this means we should evaluate students, teachers, clinical facilities, library holdings, and entire programs to determine what we do well and what we can do better so the education our students receive is the best it can possibly be. Nursing programs shouldn't be undergoing the costly, time-consuming process of NLN accreditation simply because it's "the thing to do"; they should be engaging in the process because it facilitates a critical look at our programs and improves them. Faculty shouldn't be asked to document each student's progress continually just so a complete record is on file in case the student brings legal action; they should be providing students with detailed evaluative feedback so they can develop their capabilities to practice nursing and deliver high-quality care. Additionally, faculty members shouldn't be put through the stress of being evaluated merely so there can be a piece of paper in their files; they should be evaluated to determine their strengths as teachers and as faculty members and to guide them in developing those areas where they are not as strong so their contributions to their disciplines can be valuable ones.

Of course, evaluations *are* used to make decisions about merit increases, promotions, and tenure just as evaluations are used to determine who passes a course, who is inducted into Sigma Theta Tau, and who gets an award for outstanding achievement. This aspect of evaluations cannot be denied. But faculty members should have a clear idea from their first year of employment about how well they are doing and what areas they need to develop if they want to be recommended for promotion and tenure. This guidance should come from the dean or chairperson, but it also should come from the more senior faculty members and those who hold upper ranks or are tenured. It should come as no surprise to any faculty member that she or he has not been recommended for promotion or tenure if weaknesses in performance have been identified in previous evaluations.

Maybe it's time we stepped back and looked at the *why* of evaluation before we get so anxious about the *how* or the *who*. If the purposes of the evaluation are not clear, they need to be discussed fully among all those involved in the process.

Helen, I think the fact that you have been asked to "mentor" a new faculty member attests to your chairperson's confidence in your abilities as a faculty member and her positive evaluation of you. You know what you do well and what areas you need to improve, you take student and peer evaluations of you very seriously and try to grow from them, and you continually seek feedback on your ideas, proposals, and teaching techniques. It seems to me you are more comfortable with the evaluation process than you might realize.

Maybe you need to talk about all this with the people who "hold the destiny of your career in the ink of their pens," as you put it in your letter. This should not be a secret process conducted only by members of some secret society. Evaluation is an open process, and those being "scrutinized" have the right to be involved in that process.

You know from your experience with clinical evaluation of students that it is a subjective, highly emotional process. But it is not impossible to grab hold of this "elusive butterfly" and make some sense of it for yourself. I look forward to talking with you about some of the specific issues you raised about the faculty evaluation process. Until then, try to look at faculty evaluation as comparable with clinical evaluation of students and use some of the same strategies with yourself (and your colleagues) to reduce some of the anxiety and tension associated with it. Maybe then you'll be more comfortable with the whole process and see it as a growth experience, not merely something to dread.

Good luck! Let me know how it all goes. And if you need a professional colleague to write a letter of evaluation, you know who to ask. I have a great deal of respect for your abilities as a teacher and as a faculty member, and I would be happy to share that with anyone.

13

The "Who," "What," "Where," "Why," and "How" of Faculty Evaluation

The evaluation of faculty raises questions that yield few clear answers, much like the many questions and unclear answers about the clinical evaluation of nursing students. It is a multidimensional concept, often tied to a high degree of emotionalism because it relates to rewards—tenure, promotion, merit raises, retention—and often generates a great deal of debate about who can legitimately evaluate faculty and on what criteria. If faculty members are to engage in a worthwhile evaluation process, it is essential that they examine their beliefs about evaluation and have some understanding about the various aspects of faculty evaluation.

Faculty evaluation "is intended to assist in improving the faculty member's effectiveness and in improving the quality of his work" (Ketefian, 1977, p. 718). Thus, although many faculty members perceive evaluation as a punitive, "weeding out" process, its primary purpose is assistive and growth producing in nature.

It is true that faculty evaluation "provides information on which judgments about a faculty member's general competence and thus his promotion and tenure prospects are based" (Ketefian, 1977, p. 178). If thorough, objective, constructive evaluations are conducted from the outset, however, faculty members should be well aware of their strengths and weaknesses, as well as the progress they have made in overcoming identified limitations, when promotion and tenure decisions are made. It is only when evaluations have been done in an incomplete, superficial, kind, rather than totally honest, manner, or when the feedback from previous evaluations has not been used as the basis for ongoing growth and development that unexpected promotion and tenure recommendations occur.

> An effective, systematic plan of evaluation requires commitment on the part of the faculty and administration, belief that the program is worthwhile, and belief that its value to faculty is reflected in more effective teaching and greater teacher satisfaction. (Bobbitt, 1985, p. 86)

Unfortunately, the evaluation of faculty is seen by many faculty as subjective, inconsistent, punitive, and sporadic (Centra, 1979). Flaws in evaluation systems seem to center around five major areas: (a) imprecise evaluation criteria; (b) inexplicit or poorly communicated performance expectations; (c) varying degrees of participation and involvement by those being evaluated; (d) difficulty ensuring due process for the evaluatee and legal accountability for the evaluator; and (e) little or no consideration for personal or professional values in establishing performance expectations, goals, and standards of performance.

To be most useful, all relevant dimensions of a faculty member's role must be evaluated on an ongoing basis. According to Schare (1984), classroom, clinical, and laboratory teaching each has its own set of variables, and each deserves evaluation. In fact, classroom and clinical teaching effectiveness have been studied extensively and often lie at the heart of a faculty evaluation program. What is evaluated and how it is evaluated is sometimes questioned, however.

Given the uniqueness of a *nursing* faculty member's role—particularly the aspect of clinical teaching and the extensive use of team teaching—"evaluation techniques that are designed for university-wide use cannot be used universally" (Brown & Hayes, 1979, p. 778). Classroom teaching should focus, among other things, on relationships with students, knowledge of the subject matter, and the organization and presentation of the material, and clinical teaching must be judged in relation to the activities done before, during, and after the clinical experience. Thus, the behaviors to be evaluated must be clear; in other words, a clear definition of faculty effectiveness—in all aspects of that role—is critical to a successful evaluation program (Stafford & Graves, 1978).

If a faculty evaluation program is to be effective and useful to all involved in it, it must be comprehensive, ongoing, and contributed to by many "players." Table 13.1 offers a way to visualize the many com-

Table 13.1. A Paradigm for Faculty Evaluations

The "Who"	The "What"								
	Classroom Teaching	Advisement	Clinical Teaching	Clinical Competence	Course Materials	Scholarship	Service to University	Professional Contributions	Service to Community
Students	X	X	X	X					
Nursing faculty colleagues	X		X		X	X	X	X	
Faculty colleagues in other disciplines	X				X	X	X		
External reviewers					X	X		X	
Clinical agency staff			X	X					
Administrators		X	X	X	X	X	X	X	X
Self		X	X	X	X	X	X	X	X

Note. Adapted from "A Paradigm for Faculty Evaluation" by S. Ketefian, 1977, *Nursing Outlook, 25,* pp. 718–720.

ponents of faculty evaluation. Each of the areas to be evaluated (i.e., the "what") will be described briefly, and greater attention will be given to the sources of evaluation input (i.e., the "who"). Comments on the "why" of evaluation have already been made, and those on the "where" and the "how" are integral to the following discussion.

THE "WHAT" OF FACULTY EVALUATION

Classroom Teaching

Classroom teaching evaluations should include faculty members' knowledge of the subject matter, enthusiasm about the topic, ability to encourage students to think, use of various teaching strategies, and ability to establish a positive learning environment and interactive student-teacher relationships. This list also can be expanded to include an assessment of the degree to which the conceptual framework for the curriculum is used to organize class content, the evidence of various curriculum threads (e.g., research, critical thinking), and personal mannerisms while teaching, among other criteria.

Advisement

An evaluation of faculty members' advisement responsibilities would include their accessibility to students, willingness to provide academic and career counseling, appropriate use of referrals, and knowledge of program requirements and prerequisites to provide proper guidance in program planning and course selection. In addition, such evaluations may include the extent to which advisers act as advocates for students, and the faculty members' willingness to prescribe individualized study plans for students in academic jeopardy, discuss students' feelings and emotions, and provide guidance on solving personal problems (Brock, 1978).

Clinical Teaching

Evaluating an individual's clinical teaching effectiveness must include the adequacy of all preliminary planning done with students and clinical agency staff prior to the start of a clinical experience. It also must address the appropriateness of clinical assignments given to students, the strategies used during the clinical day to help students meet objectives, the kind of challenge and support given to individual students throughout the experience, the type of relationships established with staff to create a positive learning environment for students, and the effectiveness of preclinical and postclinical conferences.

Clinical Competence

Faculty members' clinical competence must be judged in relation to their knowledge of current clinical issues and approaches, ability to demonstrate nursing interventions to students as they care for clients, clinical decision-making ability, and skill in using the nursing process. Some would argue that faculty members cannot be expected to be clinical *experts* because their primary role is teaching, not practice; however, few would argue the position that faculty members should be *competent* and comfortable in the clinical areas of practice in which they are teaching students. Indeed, Stafford and Graves (1978) addressed this latter point when they stated that students need teachers who can function well as role models, thereby demonstrating the skills, attitudes, and values that all students hope to develop.

Course Materials

An evaluation of course materials should address the clarity of the syllabus, relevance of learning experiences, and the articulation among course objectives, content, and evaluation strategies. In courses that are team taught, individual faculty contributions to the syllabus may not be discernible, but the type of test questions developed and the suggestions for updating readings and audiovisual materials used in the course often can be attributed to an individual member of the team. Course materials also should be reflective of the program's goals and conceptual framework, appropriate to the level of the students enrolled in the course, current, creative, and consistent with sound principles of teaching and learning.

Scholarly Activities

The scholarly activities of faculty members are varied and may be defined in numerous ways (Baird, et al., 1985). Typically, "scholarship" includes the following: research completed or in progress, grant proposals submitted and funded, and publications of journal articles, books, scholarly monographs, or computer programs. Presentations of papers at professional conferences—particularly papers reporting on one's own research or addressing relevant research issues—also may be included here; they are discussed further, however, in the section on professional contributions.

Service to the College or University

Perhaps one of the responsibilities that accounts for a fair portion of a faculty member's time is service to the college or university. An evaluation of contributions in this area would include the kind of department and university committees on which individuals serve, the extent to which they prepare for and contribute to such committees, their effectiveness as a committee chair, the kind of leadership they provide within their peer group, the quality with which special tasks or assignments are completed, their contributions to program recruitment activities, their cooperativeness in volunteering for or taking on assigned tasks, and the extent to which they contribute to a positive, collegial environment within the nursing department.

Professional Contributions

Professional contributions also must be considered as part of a comprehensive faculty evaluation program. As contributing members of the profession, nursing faculty members are expected to hold membership in various professional organizations, serve on committees or hold office in such organizations, and support the profession by attending and participating in conferences and workshops. Activities in this area might also include presentations made to professional groups, consultation services rendered, service on journal editorial boards, book reviews, and serving on dissertation committees outside one's place of employment.

Service to the Community

Finally, faculty frequently are evaluated on their service to the community. Activities in this area include positions on school boards, volunteer work in various organizations (e.g., Red Cross, homeless projects, American Heart Association, League of Women Voters), and service to one's religious organization (e.g., eucharistic minister, youth group adviser, church board of directors member).

It is clear, then, that the "what" of faculty evaluation is multifaceted and addresses expectations in numerous areas of performance and contribution. The other major aspect of faculty evaluation, however, is the "who."

THE "WHO" OF FACULTY EVALUATION

Student Evaluations of Faculty

> Student evaluation of faculty continues to be a thorny problem. Often, faculty feel threatened by such evaluations and question their validity and worth. (Schwab & Karns, 1986, p. 208)

Perhaps one of the most widely and commonly used methods of faculty evaluation, student evaluation of faculty is a method that is questioned and challenged by faculty and one that has "generated considerable resistance from faculty" (Norton, 1987, p. 86). The concerns about this method are many (Scriven, 1988); however, the validity of such concerns is questionable.

Faculty often question the value of evaluations that are completed by individuals who are less knowledgeable and less qualified than they are; some even perceive is at a "prestige-weakening experience" (Armington, Reinikka, & Creighton, 1972, p. 789) or an inversion of the pecking order, which is unnatural and uncomfortable to students and faculty alike. Arguments frequently arise about the weight an evaluation should carry when it is done anonymously (as most student evaluations are) and there is no opportunity to clarify or seek explanations for a particular rating.

Many faculty hold the view that student evaluations are little more than a "popularity contest," and those faculty who are nice to students, humorous, and "easy graders" are rated more positively than faculty who "push" students to achieve higher standards and are less personable. They also may believe that students use their evaluations of faculty as opportunities to retaliate for poor grades or difficulty with the library or the amount of work they were asked to do. Indeed, Cahn (1987, p. B3) noted that "the increasing use of student evaluations was closely followed by grade inflation," presumably so that students were not antagonized by poor grades and then give poor teacher evaluations.

The validity of the tools used by students to evaluate teachers, the conditions and circumstances under which students are asked to complete such tools (e.g., after a difficult examination), the explanations given to students about how their evaluations will be used, and the seemingly disproportionate significance of such evaluations in the promotion-tenure or merit increase process also are areas of concern expressed by faculty. Indeed, the use of student evaluations of teachers comes under considerable fire by many.

The validity of such criticisms must be questioned in light of repeated research findings, however. Extensive reviews of literature on the topic (Centra, 1988; Morton, 1987) show that student ratings and scales tend to be reliable, valid, and stable over time. In addition, there is a high degree of consensus among students and graduates across many studies about what constitutes an effective teacher; repeatedly, students seem to value teachers who are enthusiastic about their work, impress students as being experts in their field, are well organized, are accessible and open to students, are fair, encourage students to think, and present material in imaginative, creative ways.

Although there may be flaws in the process of using students to evaluate teaching effectiveness, one cannot deny that "in most instances, students are the only consistent observers of the instructor throughout the course of study. They are likely to know the teacher's strengths and weaknesses better than a peer or administrator who makes an occasional visit to the classroom or practicum setting" (Morton, 1987, p. 86).

If one of the goals of nursing education is to facilitate the development of students' professional skills, faculty must appreciate that inviting students to participate in the evaluation process and guiding them to complete evaluations in an objective, responsible manner can help develop selected professional skills. "As the consumers of nursing education, students can be of considerable help to faculty in improving teaching" (Armington et al., 1972, p. 792).

Perhaps faculty members would do well to value student evaluations of their teaching, design evaluation tools and procedures that will yield the most beneficial data, educate students about the significance of responsible evaluation, and use the feedback from students to grow, change, build on their strengths, and overcome their limitations. Perhaps faculty members need to recognize that students are bright people who have something to offer, that educators are imperfect people who must continue to learn and improve, and that student evaluations of teachers can be seen as a strategy to achieve multiple and varied professional goals.

Nursing Peer Evaluations of Faculty

Perhaps one of the faculty evaluation processes written about most frequently, yet one that remains quite elusive, is that of peer evaluation. Schare (1984) cited a 1975 "Statement on Teaching Evaluation" issued by the AAUP in which that organization (a) suggested that multiple measures be used for evaluating faculty and (b) stressed the importance of peer evaluation of classroom instruction.

Peer evaluation, however, must address more than just classroom teaching. One's nursing peers can legitimately evaluate most other aspects of the faculty role as well: clinical teaching, course materials, scholarship, service to the university, professional contributions, and clinical competence. In fact, faculty members' peers may be all too quick to judge them on any of these components, provided such judgments are rendered informally, verbally, or to someone else. When peers are asked to evaluate each other formally, put their comments in writing, and share personally the positives and negatives with the individual being evaluated, they become anxious and hesitant. Why?

De Tornyay (1984) recognized the reluctance peers exhibit regarding evaluating the teaching effectiveness of their colleagues. She attributed this reluctance to several factors:

1. Peer evaluation requires time, energy, and effort, none of which are available to most faculty in excess.
2. Faculty express discomfort with the difficulty inherent in

simplifying or objectifying the complex and subjective activities that comprise teaching effectiveness.

3. Peer evaluation of one's faculty colleagues is a personal process, not a detached one as is the case with judging a manuscript for publication; this personal nature of evaluation is uncomfortable for some faculty.

4. Faculty often express political and philosophical concerns: what one says about a colleague may influence one's own welfare; or the process may create suspicion and defensiveness among colleagues.

5. There is a recognition that all faculty activities should be evaluated, not just teaching effectiveness, and a question arises as to whether peers should and can do it all or only selected "pieces."

6. Faculty express concern that regular peer evaluations, using routine forms, may emphasize standardization and, therefore, result in decreased diversity in teaching.

Despite these and other concerns about peer evaluation, it persists as a valuable method of demonstrating professional accountability and teaching effectiveness. It can be a most effective method if "the rules of the game" are clear and if it is based on trust.

The evaluation of classroom teaching by one's peers should involve judgments about many areas: the preparation that was done for the class; the learning environment that was created; the way in which the physical environment was structured or used; the teaching techniques used; interactions with students in the class; the use of summarization throughout; and the accuracy, currency, comprehensiveness, and appropriateness of the theoretical content covered (Gorecki, 1977). Likewise, clinical teaching evaluation by one's peers should address the preparation that was done for the experience, preclinical and post-clinical conferences, interactions with staff and students, clinical competence, and the quality of the learning environment in terms of role modeling, and the guidance, support, and feedback given to students (Gorecki, 1977).

Peer evaluation procedures, to be most effective and least threatening to all who are involved, must be structured like those used to evaluate students. In other words, the specific criteria to be used in making judgments must be clear and made known to the individual being evaluated beforehand, the evaluation must be carried out in an objective manner, feedback must be given to the individual promptly and in a constructive fashion based on the preestablished criteria, and there must be an opportunity for the individual to discuss the evaluation with the evaluator to clarify any misconceptions or misunderstandings.

Dombeck (1986) described the peer review process used at the University of Rochester. Peer review was defined here as "an encounter between persons equal to one another in professional education, qualifications and position, in which one person's professional pursuits were examined, discussed, and critiqued by the others" (p. 188). For this faculty, where joint appointments are the norm, peer review included critiques of clinical practice, teaching, and research. The goal of peer review in this university was to improve professional standards, and it included the presentation by faculty to students and colleagues of cases and issues from their own clinical practice. This faculty group distinguished peer critique from peer support and noted that both were critical to an effective program.

Harwood and Olson (1988) also described the peer evaluation methods used at their institution. This faculty defined a "peer" as someone with "knowledge and expertise with the subject matter, accessibility to the setting, and shared clinical specialization [for clinical evaluation]" (p. 378). They used peer evaluation as a method of documenting clinical and classroom teaching effectiveness where "peers offer a critique based on their expert knowledge of the content area and teaching strategies" (p. 377). These authors noted that a critical component of the peer evaluation process is the freedom to choose one's evaluator, and that repeated observations are necessary for a fair evaluation.

Although the selection of one's own evaluator may reduce the possibility of evaluations being used in a retaliatory way, caution must be exercised with this procedure. "Peer evaluation may [become] an essentially ritualistic process" (Stafford & Graves, 1978, p. 496) if faculty members ask for their friends to do the evaluation, knowing full well that it will be positive. To avoid such pitfalls, a procedure that calls for one self-selected and one appointed evaluator, randomly selected evaluators, or the selection of a few reviewers from among several who have been assigned or randomly selected as potential evaluators may be the best solution. If the evaluation is done to help a faculty member, one should expect objective, critical feedback that points out strengths and weaknesses; one should not be satisfied only with a "pat on the back" from a friend.

It is important that faculty members clearly define what they mean by a peer: Someone who holds the same credentials, has the same rank, is or is not tenured, shares the same clinical specialty area, teaches or has taught the same courses, teaches in the same program (i.e., undergraduate or graduate), or has or has not published? Each faculty group also must describe a peer evaluation procedure that is appropriate to their size, structure, goals, and profile; additionally, that procedure must specify the following: whether peer review is required or voluntary, how evaluators are designated, when and where evaluations are completed, what is evaluated (e.g., clinical teaching, course materials), what criteria are used to make the evaluation, who reviews the evaluation, and how data are used. It is only then that many of the concerns and fears about peer review may be dispersed.

Peer Review by Colleagues in Other Disciplines

A nursing faculty member in a college or university has another group of peers who may play a role in the evaluation process, and that group is the faculty in other disciplines. Although these individuals may not be peers in terms of a background and experience in nursing, they are individuals who do have a background and experience in teaching and who are familiar with the faculty role.

Faculty colleagues in disciplines outside of nursing can legitimately provide evaluative feedback in the areas of classroom teaching, course materials, service to the university, and scholarship. Although these colleagues cannot comment on the accuracy, currency, or comprehensiveness of the nursing content presented in class, they can comment on the clarity of the presentation, its logical organization, the extent to which research and other relevant predesignated concepts (e.g., nutrition, adaptation) were integrated, teacher-student relationships and interactions, the appropriateness and effectiveness with which various teaching strategies were used, the extent to which student clinical experiences were integrated, and the ability to answer students' questions and help them think, among other things.

Colleagues in other disciplines also can review course materials and make some determinations as to the clarity of objectives, the relevance of learning experiences and evaluation methods to the course objectives, the breadth and currency of bibliographies, the "technical quality" of examinations, and so on. In addition, they can—and frequently do, as part of a tenure and promotion process—review a nursing faculty member's scholarly products; papers can be judged in terms of their provocativeness, published articles can be evaluated regarding the extent to which they reflect general scholarly standards, and grant proposals can be evaluated for their clarity and soundness. Additionally, faculty in other disciplines may be able to provide feedback on nursing faculty members' contributions to the university if they have served on committees or special projects together; such comments may be particularly valuable in that they compare nursing faculty to standards used outside their discipline.

Thus, although it would be inappropriate for peers in other disciplines to evaluate nursing faculty in the clinical area, on their advisement skills, or on their contributions to the field, they can provide valuable—and perhaps a very objective—evaluation of faculty in selected areas. De Tornyay (1984) advocated this component of comprehensive faculty evaluation plan, and nursing faculty might benefit greatly from it. In addition, faculty in other fields also may learn a great deal about nursing, the quality of nursing curricula, the excellence of nursing faculty, and the positive student-teacher relationships often enjoyed in nursing. The outcome of this could be an enhanced image of nursing throughout one's academic community, as well as growth for the faculty members who were evaluated.

Evaluation of Faculty by External Reviewers

Any nursing faculty member whose class or clinical group has been observed by a visitor during an NLN accreditation site visit is accustomed to being evaluated—in some respect—by an external reviewer. The comments written by the visitor that appear in the site visit team's report do serve as a source of feedback for that faculty member. Evaluation by external reviewers usually takes a different form, is more limited in scope, and is done for a different reason, however.

Typically, outside evaluators are called on during a tenure or promotion review to provide feedback about the candidate's scholarly contributions. External reviewers frequently share candidates' same areas of expertise, and they are asked to judge their publications in terms of their significance, value, and quality.

External reviewers also could be called on to provide feedback on the quality and importance of faculty members' contributions to the profession, the recognition afforded them by the professional community, and the way in which they have had an impact on or provided leadership in the field. As educators, they also might be asked to review course materials as previously discussed.

The individuals selected to provide an external review may be suggested by candidates, selected by the dean or department chairperson, or both. They are selected based on their own professional accomplishments and scholarship, and they can provide valuable, objective feedback on faculty members.

Clinical Agency Staff Evaluations of Faculty

Very little has been written about the use of clinical agency staff to evaluate faculty, and it would seem that few schools use this source of data. If a comprehensive, multidimensional approach to faculty evaluation is sought, however, input from this group may be deemed a necessary and valuable part of it.

In an article on problems in evaluating teaching effectiveness, Stafford and Graves (1978, p. 495) asserted a most sobering point: "The nursing faculty are the 'critical variable' in the total educational experience" of students. It would seem that this is particularly true when it comes to students' clinical experiences.

It is the faculty members, not the clinical agency staff, who must take responsibility for explaining the curriculum, the particular course in which the students on the unit are enrolled, and what can reasonably be expected of students at that level. It is the faculty members who must engage in extensive preplanning for the clinical experience and familiarize themselves with the operations of the unit, the policies of the institution, and the philosophy and goals of the nursing service department. To rely on those who arrange the overall experience—that is, the agency's affiliations coordinator and the school's department chairperson or program director—to attend to all the planning and preparatory details is foolhardy and irresponsible. The clinical agency staff can give feedback on how well faculty members have done in "laying the groundwork" for a positive experience.

In addition to input such as this, clinical agency staff can comment on the effectiveness of faculty members in promoting positive relationships among students and staff, enhancing open communications throughout the experience, and serving as a resource and guide to students during their clinical experience. Finally, although the staff cannot legitimately offer evaluative comments on faculty members' scholarly or professional contributions, they can attest to their clinical competence and ability to teach students in the clinical area.

Faculty should not feel threatened or intimidated at the thought of being evaluated by clinical agency staff. The input of nurse colleagues can be extremely helpful in sketching a more complete picture of faculty members' strengths and areas needing improvement. Provided the input they are asked to give is appropriate (i.e., focused on clinical competence and clinical teaching abilities in their broadest sense), clinical agency staff can play a most useful role in the evaluation of nursing faculty members.

Evaluation by Administrators

One of the individuals who usually can provide a valid evaluation of all aspects of faculty members' performance and accomplishments is the department chairperson, program director, or dean. This individual, as a nurse, is in a position to evaluate classroom and clinical teaching, clinical competence, and course materials. As the person who has responsibility for the nursing program, the administrator can attest to faculty members' advisement skills and service to the institution and the community. As a member of the broader nursing community, the administrator is in a position to evaluate faculty members' scholarship and professional contributions.

Faculty may want to discuss with the administrator how data will be gathered, what sources of information would be most helpful in the evaluation process, and what the expectations are for faculty. They also should feel free to discuss with the administrator any student or peer evaluations with which they take issue and how evaluation data are used. Although administrators often are "the final step" in a faculty evaluation process, they are not the only facet of that evaluation; thus, the evaluation procedures, criteria used, and feedback between faculty and administrators should be as open as they are among faculty peers and between faculty and students.

Self-Evaluation by Faculty

By far, the most comprehensive evaluation of faculty members can be provided by faculty themselves. Although such an evaluation may be the most comprehensive, however, it does not necessarily follow that it would be the most objective.

It has been noted that self-evaluations are tied to one's self-confidence; those individuals with a high confidence level tend to rate themselves higher, and those with a low confidence level often rate themselves lower (Stafford & Graves, 1978). Thus, some faculty may overinflate the significance or quality of their performance (designating every presentation as a keynote address, describing expected committee activities as extraordinary service, or listing a letter to the editor as a scholarly publication, for example). Likewise, other faculty members may not even report a major project they did for a committee because they saw that merely as a part of the expected committee work; some faculty members may not share extremely creative course material they developed because they assumed all faculty did that same type of course development and their work was not out of the ordinary.

Thus, self-evaluation, although it is an extremely important part of a comprehensive evaluation package, must not come to be viewed as the only source of evaluative input or the most significant aspect of the process. It must be balanced by other types of data. Indeed, "if self-evaluations are tempered by evaluative data from other sources, a rational perspective is likely to be maintained" (Stafford & Graves, 1978, p. 497).

SUMMARY

The evaluation of faculty is a complex, multidimensional process that should be open, systematic, and comprehensive and that should be carried out for the purpose of enhancing faculty growth, strengthening the program in which that faculty member teaches, and ultimately advancing the profession. In fact, "if faculty [is] to believe the evaluation process is effective and helpful, the data collected should serve a purpose for the individual faculty member as well as for administration" (Bobbitt, 1985, p. 88).

A comprehensive evaluation plan should provide for data to be gathered about faculty members' classroom and clinical teaching skills, course materials, clinical competence, advisement abilities, scholarship, contributions to the profession, and service to the university and community. In addition, it should provide for input from students, faculty colleagues in nursing and other disciplines, clinical agency staff, and external reviewers, as well as administrators and faculty members themselves.

Faculty and administrators should collaborate to define the purpose of faculty evaluation, the concept of peer, beliefs about student evaluations, the criteria to be used in evaluating each component of the faculty role, and the specific evaluation procedures to be followed. All faculty may be required to follow the same procedures and use the same forms, or they may have a range of options from which to select those that are best suited to reflect their achievements; this latter approach was described recently by Harwood and Olson (1988).

In addition, decisions must be made about what criteria and procedures are to be used under what circumstances. In most cases, evaluation criteria cut across ranks and are used for any number of situations. At one school, however, the faculty members developed separate performance criteria for various faculty ranks, for the program in which the individual taught (i.e., graduate or undergraduate), and for appointment, retention, promotion, or tenure decisions (Garrity, Miller, Osborn, & Vanderlinden, 1980).

Thus, the faculty evaluation plan that is developed must meet the needs of and be consistent with the beliefs of each faculty group. The implementation of such a plan would enhance teaching and promote the professional growth and development of faculty. It would also achieve a broader purpose: role modeling professional behaviors for students and helping them appreciate the value of ongoing, systematic evaluation and how a subjective process can be made more objective.

REFERENCES

Armington, C., Reinikka, E., & Creighton, H. (1972). Student evaluation — Threat or incentive? *Nursing Outlook, 20*(12), 789–792.

Baird, S. C., Biegel, A., Bopp, A., Dolphin, N. W., Ernst, N., Hagedorn, M., Malkiewicz, J., Payton, R. J., & Sawatsky, G. (1985). Defining scholarly activity in nursing education. *Journal of Nursing Education, 24*(4), 143–147.

Bobbitt, K. C. (1985). Systematic faculty evaluation: A growing critical concern. *Journal of Nursing Education, 24*(2), 86–88.

Brock, S. C. (1978, October). Measuring faculty advisor effectiveness. Paper presented at the Second Annual Conference on Academic Advising, Center for Faculty Evaluation and Development, Kansas State University, Manhattan, KS.

Brown, D. L., & Hayes, E. R. (1979). Evaluation tools: Students' assessment of faculty. *Nursing Outlook, 27*(12), 778–781.

Cahn, S. M. (1987). Faculty members should be evaluated by their peers, not by their students [Opinion]. *Chronicle of Higher Education, 34*(7), B2–B3.

Centra, J. A. (1979). *Determining faculty effectiveness: Assessing teaching, research and service for personnel decisions and improvement.* San Francisco: Jossey-Bass.

Centra, J. A. (1988). Faculty evaluation and faculty development in higher education. Unpublished manuscript.

de Tornyay, R. (1984). Evaluating teacher effectiveness [Editorial]. *Journal of Nursing Education, 23*(5), 177.

Dombeck, M. T. (1986). Faculty peer review in a group setting. *Nursing Outlook, 34*(4), 188–192.

Garrity, M., Miller, V., Osborn, M., & Vanderlinden, M. (1980). Developing criteria for promotion and tenure. *Nursing Outlook, 28*(3), 187–191.

Gorecki, Y. (1977). Faculty peer review. *Nursing Outlook, 25*(7), 439–442.

Harwood, C. H., & Olson, J. (1988). Peer evaluation: A component of faculty performance appraisal. *Journal of Nursing Education, 27*(8), 377–379.

Ketefian, S. (1977). A paradigm for faculty evaluation. *Nursing Outlook, 25*(11), 718–720.

Morton, P. G. (1987). Student evaluation of teaching: Potential and limitations. *Nursing Outlook, 35*(2), 86–88.

Schare, B. L. (1984). An appraisal process for classroom teaching in higher education. *Journal of Nursing Education, 23*(1), 40–42.

Schwab, T., & Karns, P. (1986). Decoding your student evaluations. *Nursing Outlook, 34*(4), 208.

Scriven, M. (1988). The validity of student ratings. *Instructional Evaluation*, 9(2), 5–18.
Stafford, L., & Graves, C. C., Jr. (1978). Some problems in evaluating teaching effectiveness. *Nursing Outlook*, 26(8), 494–497.

14

Faculty Evaluation as a Tool for Professional Growth

It is evident from the preceding discussion of the components of faculty evaluation that such a process is complex and multifaceted. Evaluation is intended to provide feedback to individuals and thereby assist them in improving their effectiveness and the quality of what they do. As such, the evaluation of faculty will have a significant impact on their individual professional growth and career development, the overall growth of the nursing department, and thus, the effectiveness of the nursing department in the larger university community.

VARYING EMPHASES IN EVALUATION

Because a comprehensive evaluation program incorporates several components—namely, classroom and clinical teaching, advisement, clinical competence, course materials, scholarship, service to the community and the university, and professional contributions—faculty members cannot be expected to put extraordinary effort into each area and be outstanding. Thus, at different points in an individual's career and at different phases of the nursing department's development, emphasis must be placed on selected components.

For instance, a new faculty member with no previous teaching experience may need to put more energy into the development of course materials, classroom and clinical teaching skills, and advisement skills. In this instance, the individual may have limited or no committee assignments and may not be expected to do research or to publish.

Conversely, new faculty members who have recently completed the doctorate may be encouraged to invest their energies into establishing programs of research and sharing the findings of those efforts with the nursing community through publications and presentations. In this instance, individual committee and teaching responsibility may be reduced and expected to be satisfactory, but not outstanding.

Although this course of action may seem foreign to nursing faculty who, traditionally, have valued scholarly efforts but have not allowed them to take precedence over teaching and service, it is a common practice in many other disciplines. In fact, many argue (Berry, 1989, for example) that if universities are to attract and retain scholars and researchers, these individuals must be nurtured and given the time and resources needed to develop their creative talents. Caution must be exercised, however, to avoid the extreme as outlined by Sykes (1988) where research becomes the primary concern of faculty, and teaching—particularly undergraduate teaching—advisement, course development, and participation in department and university governance becomes secondary or unimportant.

Perhaps senior nursing faculty members who have established themselves as excellent teachers and advisers as well as involved members of the department and university should be encouraged to engage in more scholarly activities or become more involved in professional organizations. Those who have made excellent contributions to the nursing department should possibly be helped to establish themselves on university committees or task forces.

Those faculty members who have had limited or no clinical teaching responsibility for several years and who wish to increase their research activities, particularly clinical research, might need to focus their energies on reestablishing their clinical competence. Those who have maintained their clinical skills and enjoy clinical teaching may need some encouragement to begin to do some research in the clinical area, perhaps in collaboration with a fellow faculty member or a colleague in the clinical agency.

In each of these instances, the area of focus for ongoing faculty activities arises out of clear faculty goals and a comprehensive evaluation that revealed the strengths for individual faculty, as well as those areas that need further development. In each instance, the individual's strengths are enhanced, and new areas of growth become the focus. Thus, the individual's career development is facilitated.

As each faculty member is supported in this way, the collective strength of the entire nursing faculty grows, and the nursing department is in a more powerful and effective position within the institution. The department can "showcase" its scholars alongside those from other disciplines. It can assure itself of a broad base of participation in significant college-wide activities. It can publicly recognize and promote the excellence of its teachers, advisers, courses, and curriculum.

CONTRACTING AND INDIVIDUAL GOAL SETTING

Although the shifting emphasis on various components of faculty evaluation is a personal matter, individuals should not make such decisions in isolation; instead, they should be made in collaboration with the program's dean or chairperson. One of the ways to do this is through individual goal setting or "contracting."

The contract faculty members receive annually (or for longer periods) is a broad agreement between the individual and the institution regarding the commitments of each: the institution agrees to employ the individual at a specific rank and pay a certain salary, and the individual agrees to fulfill the responsibilities of a faculty member. This contract does not specify *how* those faculty responsibilities are to be fulfilled or what emphasis is to be placed on each component of the role, however; thus, an individual "contract" (Aroian, Grant, & Gilbert, 1984) between faculty members and their deans or chairpersons may be in order.

Such an individualized contract may be verbal or written, and it should specify the goals and activities of the faculty member for the coming year(s). For example, one faculty member may "contract" to complete a research study in progress, submit two articles for publication on that research, submit an application for funding to build on that line of investigation, teach one graduate and one undergraduate theory course per semester, advise 10 to 15 students, and serve on one major department committee. A major focus for the designated period for individuals such as this is research and scholarly endeavors; their evaluations would give the greatest weight to success in those areas.

Another faculty member may "negotiate" to teach one undergraduate clinical and one undergraduate theory course each term; develop computer programs and other individualized learning packages to use in these courses; represent the nursing department on the university's task force on alternative teaching and learning methods; serve on the department's curriculum, learning resources, and student affairs committees; advise 15 to 20 students; serve as the faculty adviser to the student organization; and develop a proposal with an affiliating clinical agency to enhance student learning experiences and faculty practice opportunities. Individuals like this have entered into agreements where their contributions are largely in the teaching, advisement, and service domains; those areas would be weighted most heavily in their evaluations.

To meet individual and program needs, each of these types of "contracts" should be possible. Faculty members must realize, and deans must be clear to advise, however, that different options will be more likely to enhance positive promotion and tenure decisions than will others.

PROMOTION AND TENURE AS THEY RELATE TO EVALUATION

The criteria for and issues surrounding promotion and tenure were discussed in an earlier chapter and will not be reexamined here. What is relevant to explore, however, is the relationship between faculty evaluation and an individual's promotion and tenure.

The evaluations that faculty members receive throughout their "probationary" or pretenure period are invaluable in moving them toward a positive tenure review. Most universities have promotion and tenure criteria that focus on teaching (including classroom and clinical teaching, advisement, and course materials), scholarship, and service (to the university, community, and profession); however, the one that seems to weigh most heavily in such decisions in senior colleges and universities today is that of scholarship

As universities look to enhance their reputations, secure government and private funding, and attract scholars and experts in various disciplines, the emphasis on scholarship is growing in most universities. As nursing strives to develop its scientific base and establish its credibility and position in the larger community of scholars, this emphasis is growing in many nursing academic units as well (Baird et al., 1985). New faculty members, therefore, would be wise to discuss these trends with their chairpersons and then to negotiate individualized contracts that will help them develop in this area. The example given earlier about the faculty member who negotiated to focus on scholarly activities would probably be in a better position to be reviewed positively for tenure in a senior college or university than would faculty members who contracted to focus on teaching and student activities. It must be noted, however, that if the latter individuals were already tenured, they should be permitted to develop and refine these areas and be evaluated accordingly.

In most academic settings, it is presumed that one is at least satisfactory, if not excellent, as a teacher by the time one is reviewed for tenure. It also is usually presumed that the individual has contributed at least satisfactorily to the profession and the department (and perhaps to the institution and community) by that time. Some (Watkins, 1985) assert, however, that "outside activities," which "utilize a professor's expertise in his or her academic discipline" (p. 23), should not be glossed over too quickly because they also enhance the university's reputation and strengthen the relationship between the university and various communities.

In addition, most colleges and universities have no mechanism for recognizing or considering one's clinical competence because, despite nursing and other fields being practice based, one is employed by an academic institution to be a teacher and a scholar, not a clinician. Indeed, the clinical nature of nursing raises questions regarding faculty evaluation that other disciplines do not face (Stafford & Graves, 1978). Nursing faculty must work to change the system if they wish to see clinical practice recognized. Thus, in many schools, all these areas are not weighted as heavily in tenure and promotion decisions as is scholarship.

SUMMARY

The comprehensive evaluation of faculty is an important process to enhance the personal and professional development of the individual.

It also serves to promote and advance the department in which the individual teaches.

As a mechanism to promote growth and career development, evaluation and feedback must be individualized to allow for various emphases of efforts, but it also must be related to the overall goals of the department. Thus, individualized contracting (or some variation thereof) between the chairperson and a faculty member for promotion and tenure reviews, enhance the position of the department in the university, and provide the basis for individual faculty evaluations and merit raises.

Faculty members need not fear the process of evaluation. Instead, they should view evaluation as an opportunity to receive feedback about their strengths and limitations, and use evaluation data as a means to guide and enhance their career development. It is only then that they will become "a force to be reckoned with" within the academic community and serve as positive professional role models for their students.

REFERENCES

Aroian, J., Grant, K. J., & Gilbert, J. P. (1984). Contracting for growth. *American Journal of Nursing, 84*(8), 1042–1043.

Baird, S. C., Biegel, A., Bopp, A., Dolphin, N. W., Ernst, N., Hagedorn, M., Malkiewicz, J., Payton, R. J., & Sawatsky, G. (1985). Defining scholarly activity in nursing education. *Journal of Nursing Education, 24*(4), 143–147.

Berry, E. (1989). Newly hired young scholars should be nurtured, not resented [Point of view]. *Chronicle of Higher Education, 35*(41), A36.

Stafford, L., & Graves, C. C., Jr. (1978). Some problems in evaluating teaching effectiveness. *Nursing Outlook, 26*(8), 494–497.

Sykes, C. J. (1988). *ProfScam: Professors and the demise of higher education.* Washington, DC: Regnery Gateway.

Watkins, B. T. (1985). Colleges urged to weigh professors' outside activities during evaluations for salary increases and tenure. *Chronicle of Higher Education, 31*(12), 23–24.

Index

Index